To Gene
all the Best

Ben Johnson
1007
4.79

Seoul to Soul

AUTOBIOGRAPHY

BY BEN JOHNSON JR.

Ben Johnson

www.benjohnsonenterprises.com

*Judge not, and ye shall not be judged;
condemn not, and ye shall not be condemned;
forgive, and ye shall be forgiven...*

Luke 6:37
(King James Version)

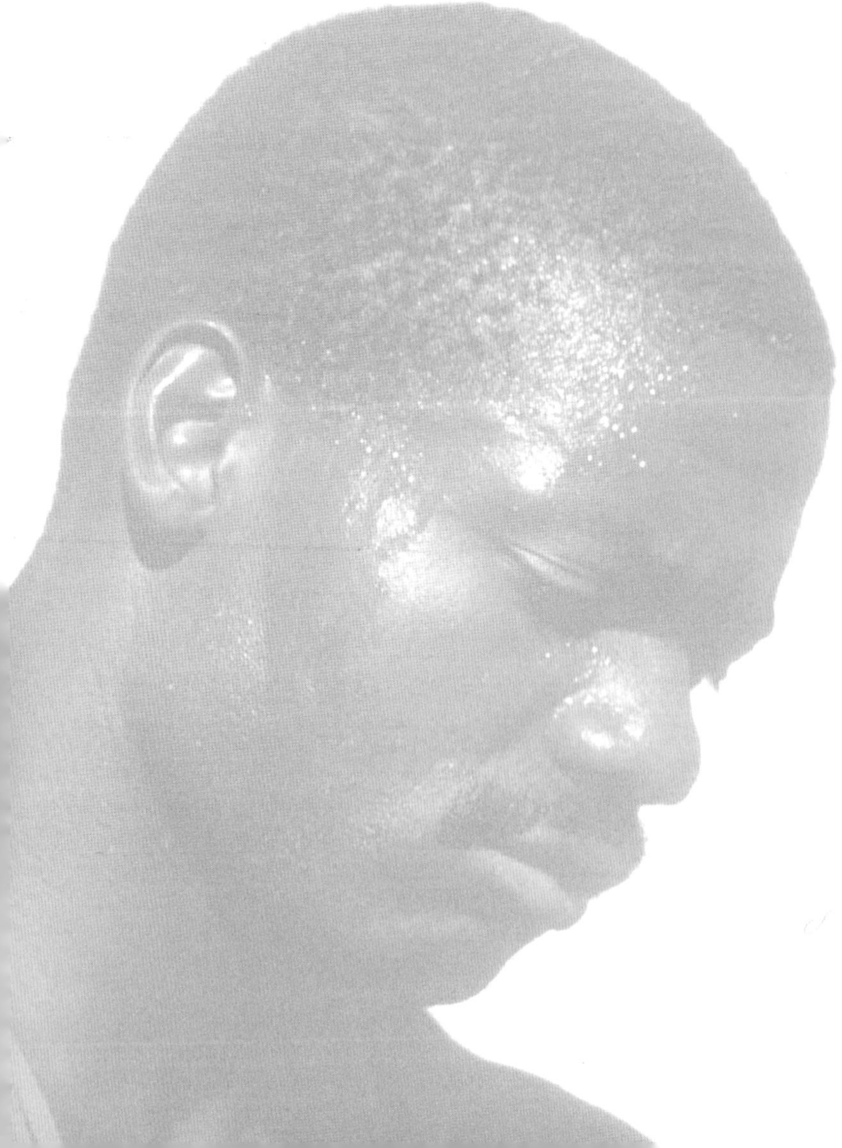

D E D I C A T I O N

For My Mother

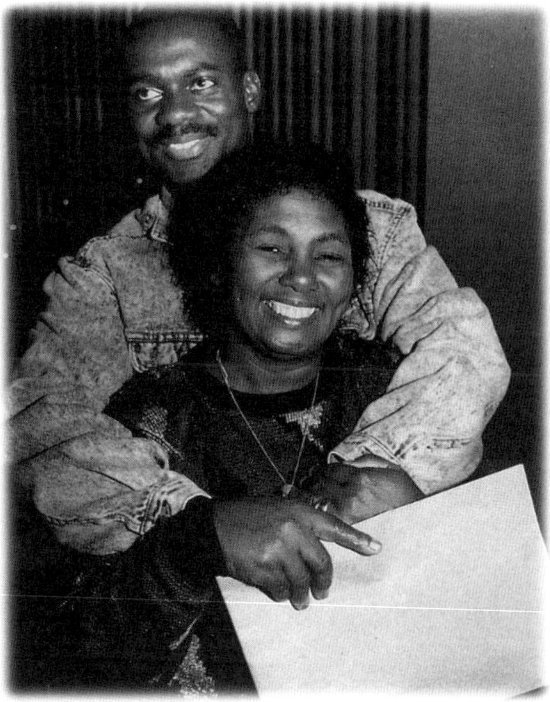

Gloria Melrose Johnson

1935 - 2004

FIRST EDITION

http://www.benjohnsonenterprises.com

ISBN 978-0-9865077-0-0

UPC 627843093473

Seoul to Soul

Special thanks to my writing and editing team:
Jill E. Meyer, Dianne MacDonald and Catherine Allen
and to all other contributors.

And special thanks to
Bryan Farnum
and his team at Blunt.fm Truth Radio,
who can be reached at www.blunt.fm.

Printed in Canada

APPRECIATION

I shall never forget to acknowledge that without God's Divine intervention, I would not have had the opportunity to publish this book nor experience all that life has presented to me. I thank God and I give all the glory to God. The last thing I need is for others to worship me. I will remain humble to my last breath.

Thank you to all who were brave enough to come forward and provide me with information I needed and to everyone who worked diligently to complete this book. I am grateful to my spiritual advisor, Bryan Farnum, for deep Truths revealed through his powerful gift of discerning God's Truth. Without these discernments, this book could not have been so compelling and truthful. I thank Bryan for being a vessel to assist in my ongoing healing. The cleansing of my soul is priceless to me.

TABLE OF CONTENTS

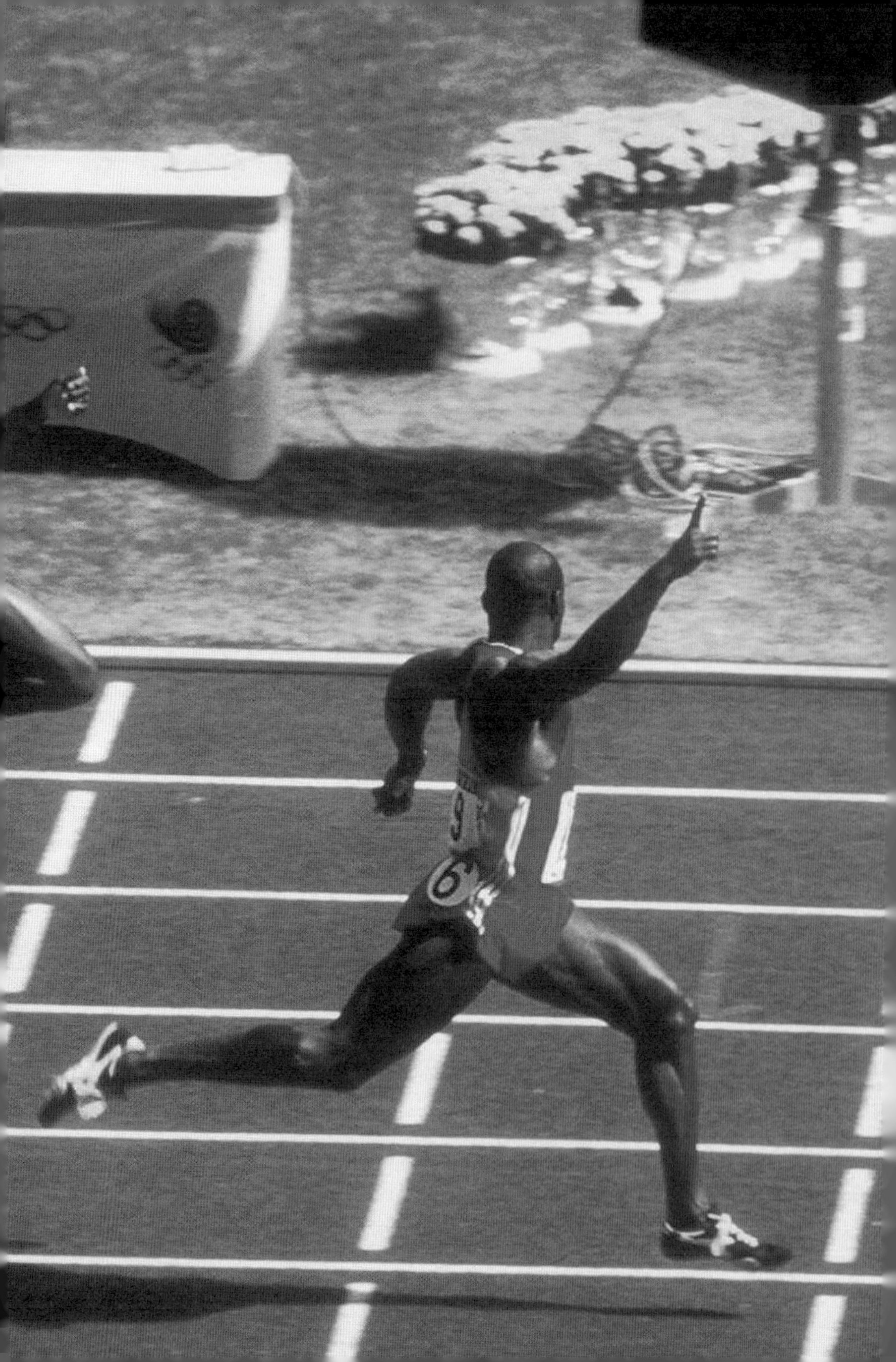

P R E F A C E

The Finish Line

Seoul, South Korea, September 24, 1988. A beautiful day. I got up early to a clear sky. The sun was out. As I looked up from my balcony that morning, I prayed. I asked for protection and guidance. I also asked that God's Will be done, knowing whether I won the gold medal or not, I would still be happy in God's Hands.

Here I am... running. The finish line is coming. When I am through, there will be nothing left. There will be nothing left in the tank, only fumes, fumes enough to run a victory lap, maybe only half. When I am through, there will be only me. Here is where I will lay it all out, holding nothing back. Here, there is only me. There is no one else. I hear... but there is no sound. I see... but there is nothing ahead, only empty space, which I will fill with my speed. I am wind. I am air. I am the bullet from a gun. I fly, I don't run. I am at 80 metres now. Mom, can you see me? Dad, can you see me? I made it. I made it through! I came through! I am ahead, not behind. I am out in front! I am the winner. And I thank God! I will raise my hand to celebrate for you, Mom, Dad and God. I salute you. A job well done. Thank you. And thanks to all my fans. It was a great run and an excellent race.

Twenty-two years later, I asked my spiritual advisor, Bryan Farnum to ask God, "Even though I prayed, why was I not protected?"

Bryan sat back in his chair, closed his eyes, and began discerning* the Truth. He surrendered himself to God. With the frequency of love in his voice, Bryan spoke to my heart, but I knew it was not him speaking. I knew it was God speaking through Bryan, answering my question:**

Ben, for did I not give you your mother as the vessel to protect you? Did she warn you not to accept food or drink from a stranger? My son, I did protect you, for the amount of steroids that were in your body might have taken your life.

*To discern means to serve as a vessel, allowing the Christ, the Spiritual Body of God, to flow through and express Truth.

**Editor's note: For the remainder of this book, all discernments provided by Bryan, serving as a vessel to deliver God's Words, will appear in *italics.*

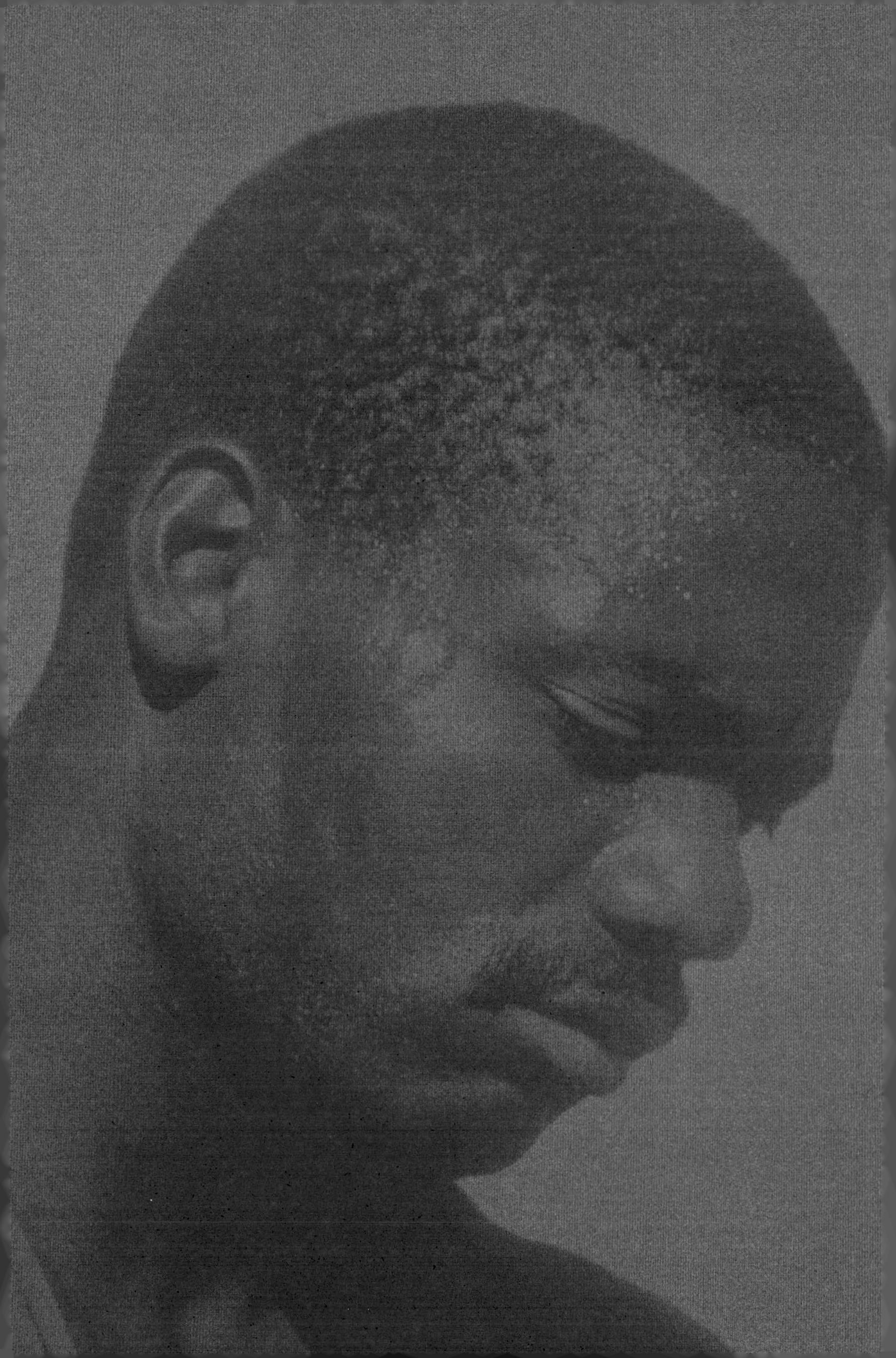

CHAPTER 1

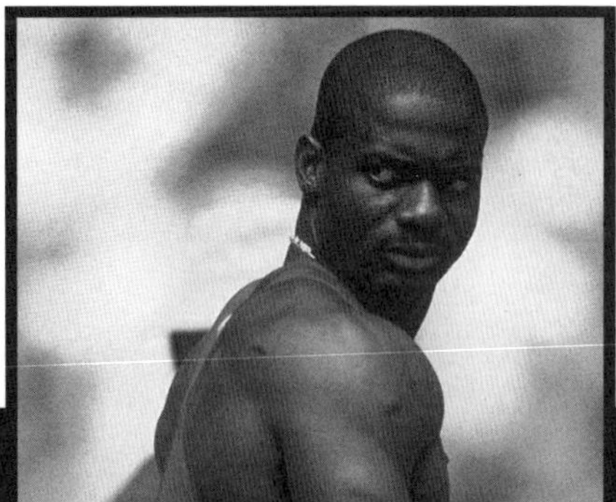

Winning the Race but Losing My Medal

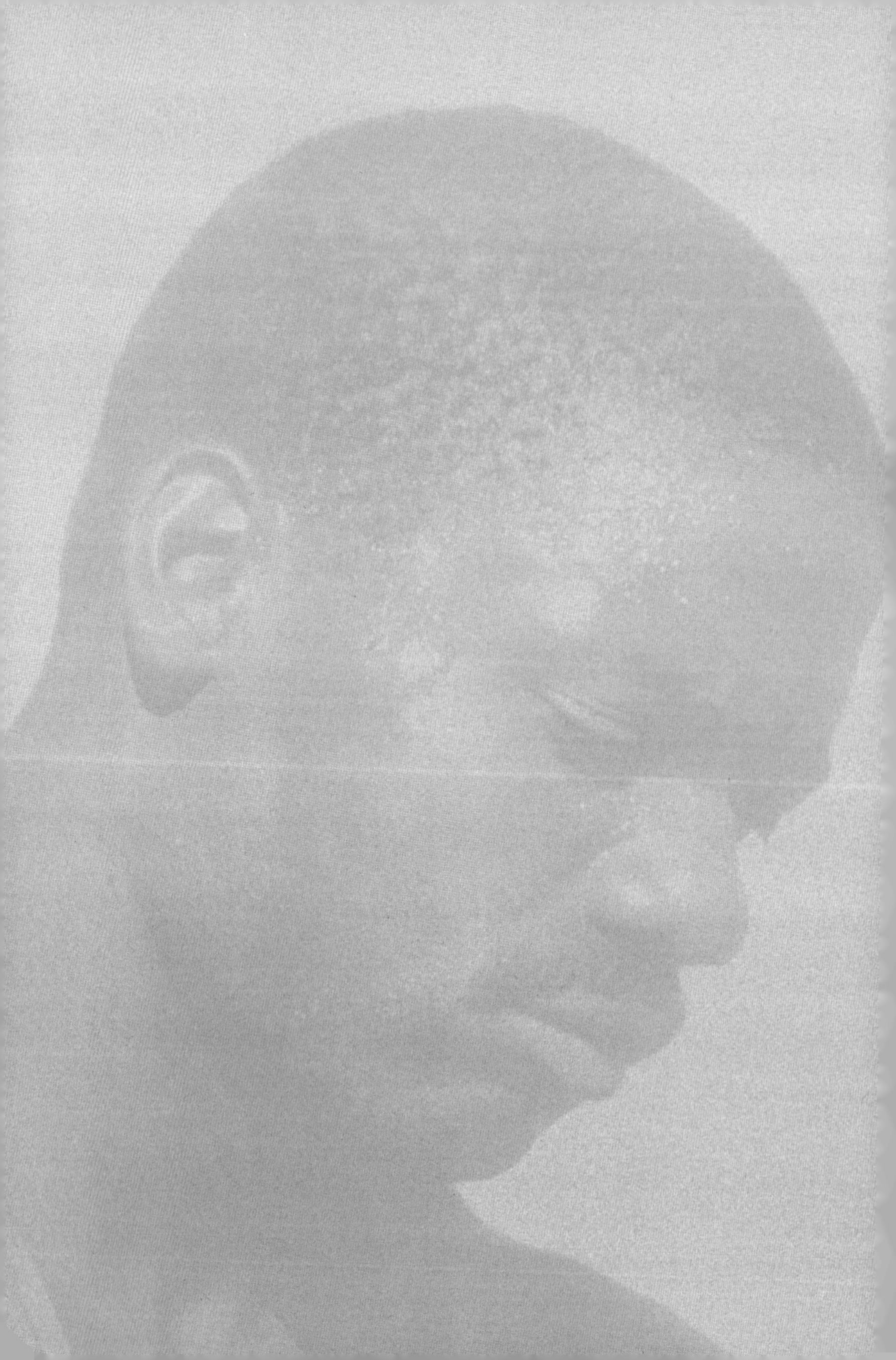

CHAPTER 1

Winning the Race but Losing My Medal

Normal protocol seemed to follow my race in Seoul. Two Olympic officials escorted me off the track to the doping testing area to wait for a member of the IOC. Before I could actually make it into the room reserved for the winner of the 100 metre race, an official with the Canadian Olympic Association, Diane Clement, approached me. She said the Prime Minister of Canada, Brian Mulroney, wanted to talk to me and CBC wanted to interview me. Only at this point was I able to see my coach, Charlie Francis, and my agent, Larry Heidebrecht, in the hall. We happily grabbed each other and hugged in passing. Officials told me that someone from the IOC would have to accompany me everywhere I went until I gave my urine sample. So Diane, one of the doping officials and I all went together to the CBC booth upstairs, where I spoke to Prime Minister Mulroney. He told me he and his family had watched the race and it was a very proud day for Canada. He wanted to offer his

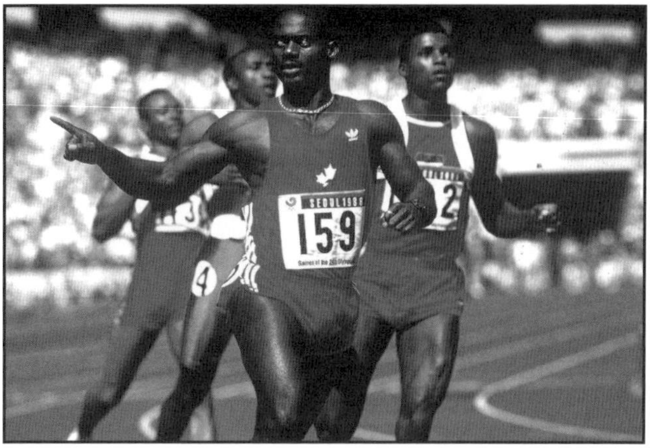

personal congratulations. I finished the interview with CBC and then the doping official escorted me back to the testing area.

There were a lot of people around the testing area, including athletes from other countries who had just completed their events. We were all waiting to get tested, with the exception of one person. I could not understand why he was there. He did not win any event. In fact, he had not even competed. I knew him. He was André "Action" Jackson, a man whose path had crossed with mine several times, a man who was also a good and long-time friend of Carl Lewis. Today, Dr. André "Action" Diakité Jackson or M'Zée Fula-Ngenge, as he is more commonly known, is the head of JFPI Corporation, Africa's largest holding company.

When I was brought to the doping control waiting room reserved for the gold medalist, André was already inside the room. He approached me to congratulate me. There was a bench in the room. I needed to lie down and have Waldemar Matuszewski, my physio- and massage therapist, work on my Achilles while I waited until I could provide my urine sample.

The IOC had equipped every room with a refrigerator stocked with an assortment of drinks. André opened the fridge, pulled out a cold beer, and offered it to me. I was not in the habit of drinking alcohol. But after all, it was a time for celebration. So, I just accepted André's offer as a kind gesture: I didn't think much more of it at the time.

Interestingly, I had made a request earlier to have Charlie and our team doctor, Jamie Astaphan, join me in the doping room. But the officials denied my request. According to the officials, Charlie and Jamie did not have security clearance to come in. Meanwhile, André, who did not seem to have any real purpose in being there, made himself at home in the doping room. He was sitting down on the floor beside the refrigerator, and grabbed and opened another can of beer. Again, I thought nothing of it when he offered me a second beer. I was very thirsty, not to mention in pain, and so, I guzzled it down just like I did the first. I really wanted to get out of there and begin to relax and enjoy my victory. I stayed in the doping room for more than three hours. During this time, I must have had about eight beers.

Carl Lewis was in a room adjacent to mine. I did not notice him at first and, as always, I was not expecting any acknowledgement from him. But to my surprise, he seemed relaxed and at ease. He was well-known to me, as well as to other racers, as a sore loser. But that day, he appeared to be in a good mood. His calmness appeared to me to be an unusual response. In Jamaica we say, "You shake man han', you nuh shake 'im heart." With Carl, I could never tell for sure what was going on. What you saw on the outside was not always the same on the inside. But by then, the beers were having an effect on me. I didn't care very much.

When I think about it now, it still amazes me how so many people had access to my waiting area. During the course of the three hours, a lot of people entered my room. In addition to various Olympic officials and André, some African athletes and their coaches also stopped by my room. Yet security measures did not allow Charlie and Jamie to be with me. Meanwhile, it appeared that André had access to wherever he wanted to go.

Photographers came in and out. Some pictures were taken of the two of us, André on the floor and me on the bench, lying prone and propped up on my arms. Diane Clement came in and André and I had our picture taken with her, too. Then, André got up and left the room. I was relieved when the doping assistant showed up to take me down the hallway for my test.

As I left my waiting room, I could hear Carl and André talking and laughing very loudly. When my eyes caught theirs through the doorway to Carl's room, they froze. Carl gave me a strange smile that I never forgot. For 20 years after that moment, I often wondered what that smile meant. I often wondered if it indicated that he knew about the plot to sabotage me. I wondered if he was nervous. What did he know?

Years later, after I met my spiritual advisor, Bryan Farnum, I asked him to discern* why Carl was smiling. Bryan has a very powerful spiritual gift to discern all levels of God's Truth on a yea, yea; nay, nay basis. Through his gift, Bryan is allowed access to God's Spiritual Archives. These Archives contain vast amounts of information on

*To discern means to serve as a vessel, allowing the Christ, the Spiritual Body of God, to flow through and express Truth.

everything and everyone, all of God's Truth. With God's permission, Bryan can access any individual's file in order to help them. Bryan's purpose is to serve as a vessel of God's Truth, bringing people together, providing His Truth to facilitate healing and forgiveness. As a Messenger of God, he is able to surrender himself to God so that God's Words can come through him. When I hear the frequency and vibration of Bryan's voice, it strikes a chord in my heart and I know the Truth is touching my soul. God spoke to me through Bryan, answering my question:*

Ben, a smile can mean so many things... reflections of many hallways... reflections of many different paths. For the answer remains deep. For when many have fear of losing something, many will smile. But you must remember, as you are going through a life lesson, so is Carl Lewis. Just as you are My child, Carl Lewis is My child. I ask that you do not judge Carl Lewis or find fault in Carl Lewis... as what you find with Carl Lewis, if you were to judge Carl Lewis, you will always find the same within yourself. For it is better to forgive and let go of the past.

I reflected on this Message. The Father is right. As I walk on the path of healing my soul, I find I need to forgive many people. I do forgive Carl Lewis. And I ask him to forgive me.

After I finished the doping test, I just wanted to see my mother and sister. They had been in the stands watching me. Security advised me this was not possible: due to the media mayhem in the stadium, my mother and sister had been taken directly back to our hotel. I could see them there.

The testing procedure requires winners to provide a urine sample after their race. The sample is then divided in two: an "A" sample and a "B" sample. As I understand it, no names are associated with the samples at this stage of the procedure. Instead, an assigned number or code identifies them. This way, the testing labs are prevented from knowing whose urine they are testing. This anonymity is intended to make the process fair.

*Editor's note: For the remainder of this book, all discernments provided by Bryan, serving as a vessel to deliver God's Words, will appear in *italics.*

The numbers are crosschecked later with a list of names held elsewhere by the IOC's Medical Commission. Back in 1988, it was held by Prince de Mérode. If the "A" sample tests positive, then the list is checked to determine the athlete's identity. At this stage, an official finding is not confirmed unless sample "B" also tests positive.

Regardless of the official protocol for lab testing, whether it's "A" or "B," I know in my heart that the security entrusted with handling my urine sample at the Seoul Olympics did not hold any integrity. Furthermore, if a thorough investigation was conducted into today's Olympic testing procedures, we would find that the security still has no integrity. It is entirely possible for the innocent to be set up from behind the scenes. I strongly believe policies and procedures for drug testing at Olympic events should come under heavy scrutiny, so that what happened to me does not happen to anyone else.

When I finally made it back to my hotel, my mother and sister were in the lobby, waiting excitedly to congratulate me. We all went back to my room, where I sat down on the sofa, took a deep breath and said, "It's all over. I need a two-year vacation." My mother hugged me and told me she was very proud of me.

The next day, Sunday, I slept in. I took it easy that day. I went over to the stadium for a couple of hours to watch a few events with my mother, my sister and Carol Anne Letheren, the Canadian Team's Chef de Mission. I felt very good about winning the gold medal and I was looking forward to going back home to Canada to celebrate with everyone, particularly my family.

Monday morning, around 7:00 a.m., I heard a knock on my hotel room door. It was Charlie. He did not look well. Before I could even utter a word, he told me my "A" sample had tested positive for stanozolol. I was shocked and dumbfounded. I thought, "It can't be true!" These test results were bizarre, unbelievable. The thought occurred to me, "They made a mistake." I knew I did not use stanozolol before my race. Then I thought, "Maybe I have been set up... If so, they finally got me."

Today, as I look back, it still disturbs me that Carl Lewis, and the others who supported Carl, expressed no plainly observable disappointment about Carl losing the race to me, prior to the public announcement that I had tested positive. What did he know that I did not? My memories of Carl losing a race are always of him expressing great disappointment. In this case, after our race in Seoul, he did not. For years after that day, I often wondered if Carl or someone connected to him had set me up.

The test results were unbelievable. In complete shock, I called my mother who was staying in the suite next to mine. She came over immediately and without saying anything to me, she began to pray. We were all very frantic, but knew we had to act right away. Charlie and I tried to figure out what could have happened and what our next step should be. We were sure there was a mistake and once the "B" sample was tested, I would be cleared.

Hurriedly, I packed a travel bag with all the vitamin and mineral supplements I was taking. Charlie and I then rushed over to the IOC lab. We met Professor Arnold Beckett, a member of the IOC's Medical Commission. He was one of the main officials responsible for drug testing at the Olympics and was also head of the School of Pharmacy at the University of London. We showed him everything in my travel bag. He was at a loss to explain the positive results if all I had been taking was in my travel bag.

Of course, the officials and technicians connected to the IOC lab have no proof whether or not I removed any steroids from my bag. But I know for certain in my heart and soul that I did not use steroids or have any steroids in my possession during the Seoul Games. I did not know it at the time when my positive test results came back, but today, I know without doubt, the cans of beer Mr. André Jackson handed to me in the doping room were tainted with steroids.

If I had actually had stanozolol in my system when I ran the 100m final, it would have made me run a lot slower, not faster. In addition, Professor Beckett, who has since passed away, told Charlie and me the amount of steroid found in my system was actually a lethal dose. Lethal! It was hard not to think that some form of treachery was involved here.

Meanwhile, even before my "B" sample was tested and before there was an official announcement, news had already gotten out and the press was all over it. Someone had leaked the news. My fate was sealed. I was already declared guilty in public, before an official confirmation, before a positive test from my "B" sample was completed and reported. The details of my "A" sample were already big news, despite the fact that an official finding had yet to be declared. To me, this further suggested foul play was involved. How would the media have known it was my urine sample that was tainted? Who would have told them? Could they have been told this was going to happen even before it occurred? And if they knew it was my sample, why didn't they report that the level of stanozolol found could have killed me? In any case, it now seemed unlikely I was going to get a fair shake.

We returned to the hotel dejected. While we were held up in my room, the media were already in pursuit of the story surrounding my positive results. The hotel acted with speed, providing security officers to guard my door, as well as the hotel lobby where journalists and photographers had already gathered. For hours we waited. We sat restlessly, throughout the day and into the evening, waiting for the results of the "B" sample.

Finally, at 9:00 p.m., there was another knock on the door. It was Carol Anne Letheren and Dr. William Stanish, the Chief Medical Officer for the Canadian Olympic Association. The news they brought was discouraging. My "B" sample tested positive. We talked to everyone who would listen, simply trying to make an appeal. We petitioned Carol Anne, Dr. Stanish, and Jean Charest, Canada's Sports Minister, as well as Dick Pound, the IOC's Vice President, asking that the matter be investigated further. Although there were many questions regarding the security in the testing area, their response was unequivocally, "No." Flat out, "No."

According to IOC officials, they also measured my natural hormone levels, compiling an endocrine profile. From this profile, they concluded I had been using steroids for some time prior to the Olympics. On this basis, they rejected my appeal. I realize that the IOC and the IAAF were trying to do their best under the circumstances. It was difficult for all of us. This being said, to my knowledge, these profiles were never used to judge anyone else in Seoul but me, even though other athletes had tested positive in Seoul. While I don't blame the IOC for its diligence in catching performance enhancement, it seemed as though there was something unjust in how the rules were unequally applied to me. The way the whole thing unfolded in Seoul, I could not help but feel I was deliberately singled out.

The truth remains, if the beer that André Jackson gave to me had not been tainted with stanozolol, there would have been no issue with the IOC. The issue at hand is this fact: the only reason my urine sample tested positive is because I unknowingly drank tainted beer after my race. And with that, my victory was snatched from me. Everything I had worked 11 years for and accomplished two days prior had now become invalid and was wiped out of the record books.

It seemed like my family was in mourning. My mother and my sister were in tears, as if someone had died. Their sobs were heart breaking. Holding back my own tears, I told them no one had died. And I tried to console them. I can still to this day hear their cries, "Oh God." Charlie was also upset and distraught. He believed in me and he did his best to protect me. Jamie and Larry were going through their own mixed emotions.

Reflecting back, I now realize that Jamie did not outwardly appear especially shaken by the fact I had lost my gold medal. From time to time, I have wondered why. I also remember Jamie telling me prior to the actual race in Seoul that I could test positive. Just around this very same time, Jamie asked me for $1 million in compensation. We got into a big disagreement. I was very angry with Jamie and threatened to fire him after the Olympics.

I asked Bryan, "Did Jamie know ahead of time that someone would sabotage me? Did he know that André Jackson would plant steroids in my beer?" Bryan came back very quickly with the response, "For what lies in the shade shall one day be revealed in the Light."

At about 10:00 p.m., Carol Anne and Dr. Stanish returned. They had come to take back my gold medal. It was a very emotional moment for everyone present. Unable to contain herself, Carol Anne began crying, too. I could tell they all felt sorry for me. I was tired. I had been through enough. Dr. Stanish asked me for the medal. It was in my carry-on bag. I opened my bag, removed my gold medal and handed it to him. He took it. Right after I won the medal, my intent was to offer it as a gift to my mother. More than anyone else, she deserved it. But this was not meant to be. Now I had to give it back. The next day, my gold medal would be awarded to Carl Lewis.

Many tried to convince me that losing my medal was not a big deal. On a personal level, through my faith and through the influence of my mother, I knew I could overcome this, and I knew one day my family name would be cleared. I just knew it. However, to lose my gold medal was more than a big deal. It was a huge deal. Many fans worldwide trusted and believed in me. But beyond my control, I was set up to let them all down. This is the part that really hurt me the most: that I won the gold medal and then lost it, so I was unable to fulfill my life-long dream. My ultimate dream had always been simply to please my mother. I asked Bryan to discern whether or not this was true. He confirmed that it was.

The pain of this deep hurt and disappointment has since been released from my soul by certain Truths being revealed to me on a very deep spiritual level. Knowing these Truths allowed me to forgive all. But the memory is still there, the memory of how I disappointed so many. Regardless of the facts, the accountability has to be with me, particularly when my mother, a Christian and spiritually gifted person, had forewarned me many times that I must be careful when someone offered me food or drink. She always said this was the only way anyone could bring me down. Especially when we were in Seoul, she reminded me often and even went so far as to tell me not to eat at the same place twice. But at that moment in Seoul, in the doping room, when the beer was handed to me, I did not remember my mother's advice. I ask all those who trusted in me to please forgive me.

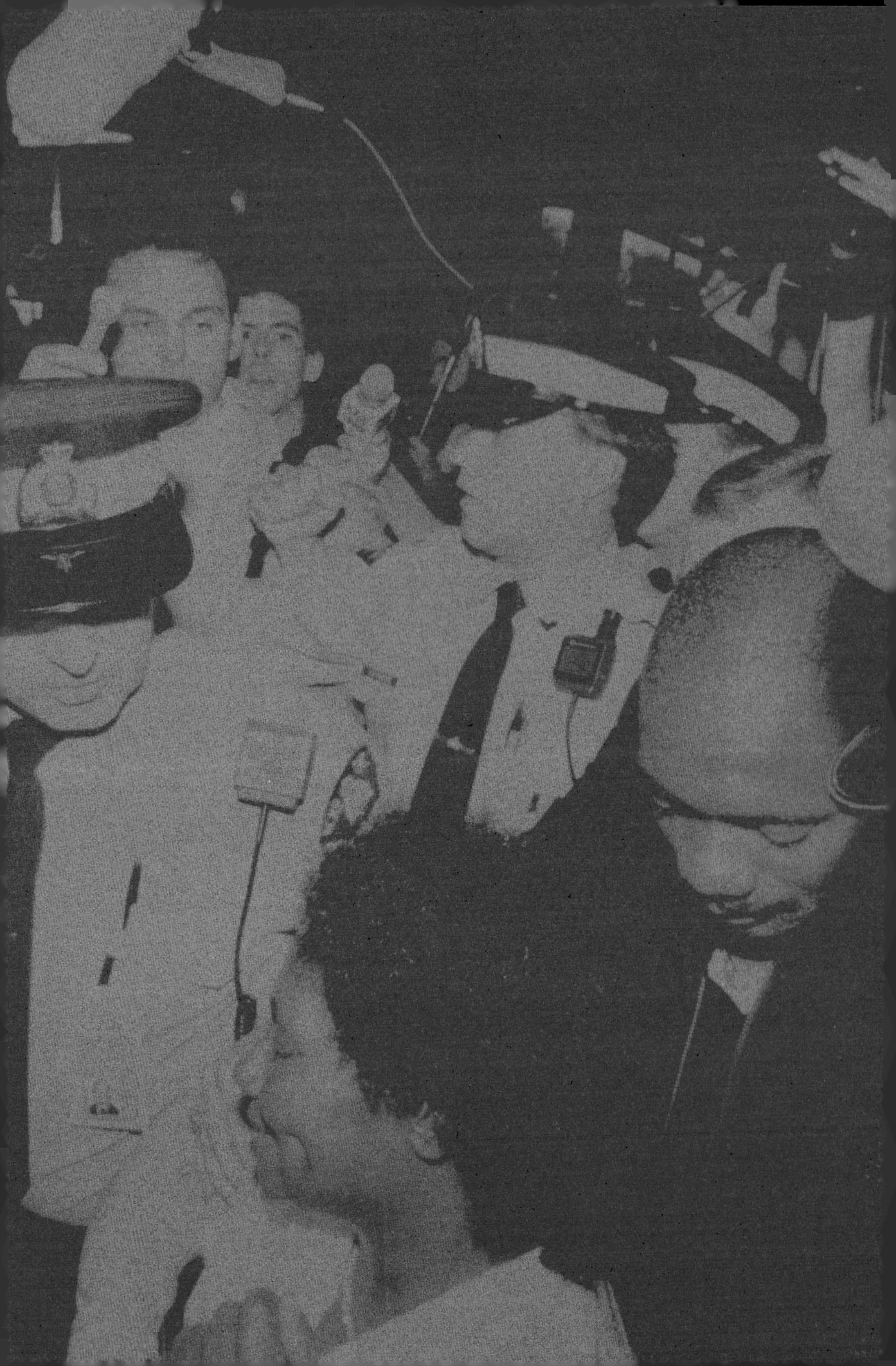

CHAPTER 2

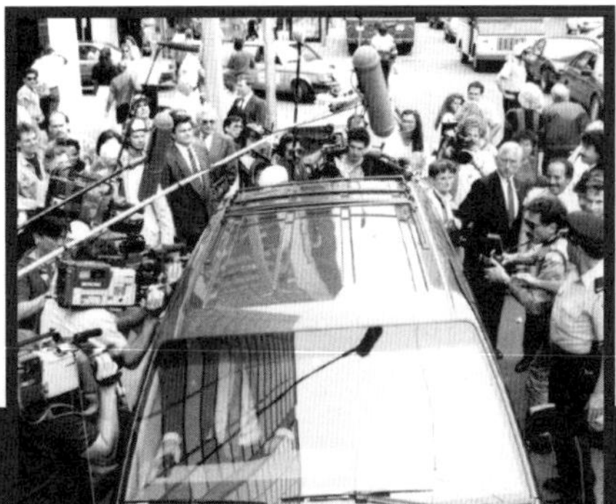

What Happened?

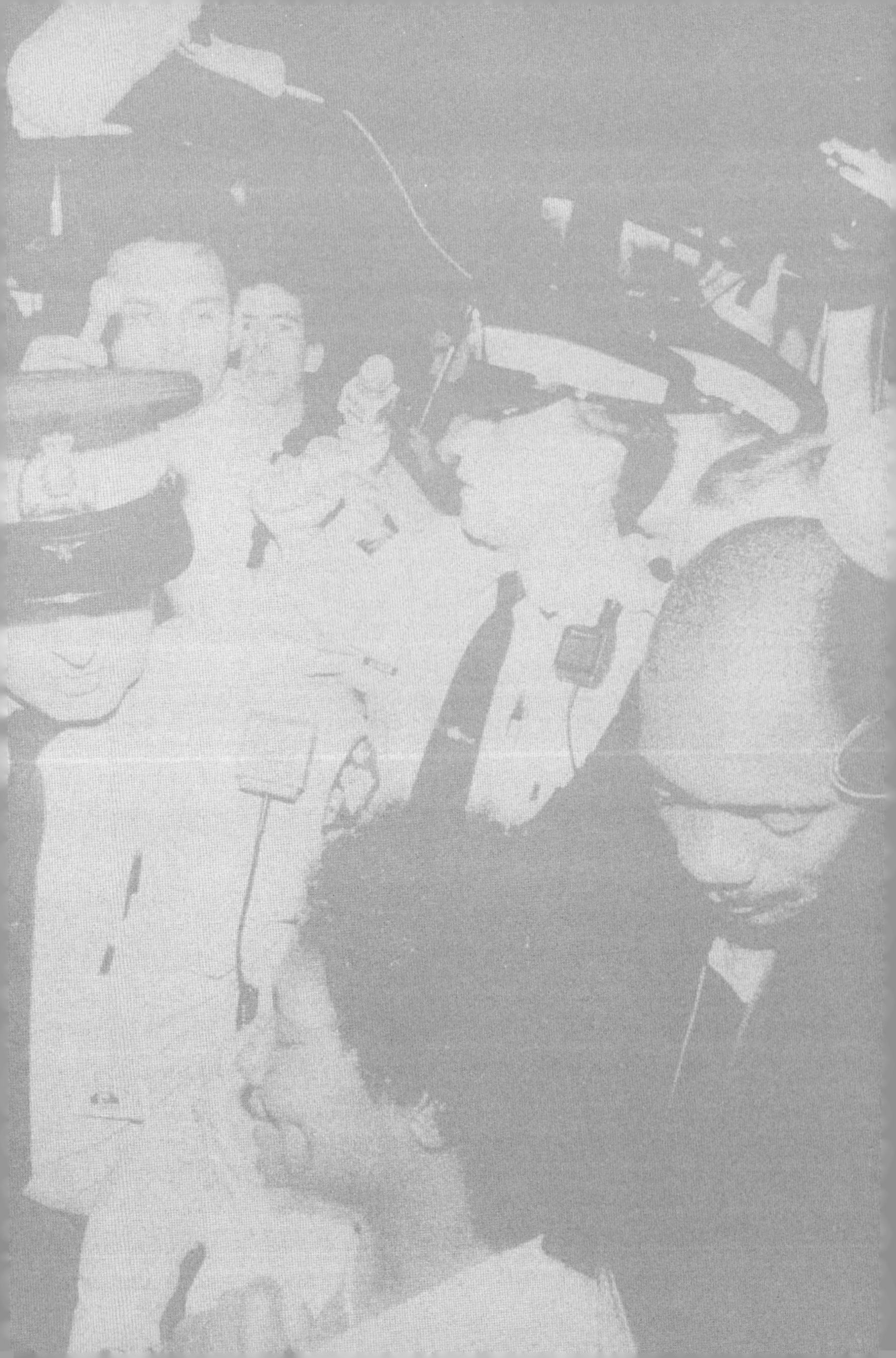

CHAPTER 2

What Happened?

A journalist once asked me during an interview to describe what I felt was taken away from me as a result of my positive test in Seoul. There was not much to say. I simply remarked, as I stared down at my body, "Well, I am still alive. And I have both my hands and feet. I am still black and I have my family. I don't feel they took anything from me." My life was not ruined after Seoul. But rebounding from the scandal was one of the hardest things I have ever had to do. Without a doubt, the following years were the toughest of my life, and of my career, to that point.

After a couple of days of unsuccessfully arguing our case and trying to convince the IOC that my positive test results warranted further investigation, we decided to leave Korea. It seemed no one with any decision-making power was willing to act on my behalf. It seemed there was not anything anyone could do. While many close to me were anxious to argue my case, I tried to remain calm and hopeful. After all, there had been other athletes who had tested positive before, only to have the decision reversed or overturned. So why would I be any different? However, when all of our appeals were rejected, I realized this part of my life as a respected Olympian was quickly coming to an abrupt halt. But I never lost my hope and I hung onto the words of my mother. She always said the truth would come out but she would not be here to see it. She maintained that everything eventually would work out. I believed her. I knew I was innocent. I knew something went terribly wrong but at that time, I did not know precisely what or exactly how.

In the midst of it all, I retreated to the safety of my family and found some peace while everything fell apart around me. Escaping the media proved to be a full-time job. They were looking for answers from me, which at that time, I did not have. Our departure from Seoul was dramatic to say the least.

Accompanied by a security detail of 50 officers, my family and I were scurried through Kimpo Airport. The flight was tense. Suspicions were strong. I was seated in first class. My mother and sister were with me. It was very overwhelming. The flight seemed to last forever. The flight attendants and passengers alike persistently wanted my autograph or their picture taken with me. The irony did not escape me. Here I was, my life seemingly crumbling and having to pose and smile for everyone else's pleasure. I sorely needed to rest. I was mentally drained.

At one point during the flight, I questioned Jamie, my doctor. I bluntly asked him what had happened. He said he did not know. I asked him if he had given me anything he was not supposed to. He said no. Today, I still wonder if Jamie influenced, to some degree, the course of events that lead to my disqualification. Was part of Jamie disappointed because he was my doctor and not Carl's? All these years later, I believe in my heart Jamie would have preferred to be Carl's doctor and his loyalty was to Carl.

Back then, deep down I could not help but wonder if my own people had betrayed me. Were they acting in my best interests? Were they motivated out of spite or greed? Why would they want to hurt my career? This did not make sense. After all, Diadora, my sponsor, had promised everyone in my entourage a new house and a large sum of cash if I won the gold medal.

Outwardly, I kept calm, but inside I was tormented by many unanswered questions. Were Charlie, and others close to me, doubting me as well? I know Charlie was heartbroken. I could not have made it this far without him.

I knew I had let many people down from the response of the media and many close to me. It certainly was agonizing for me, too. I simply could not fathom that I was going through this experience. I could not comprehend losing my gold medal. If I had known in my heart that I actually took the steroids I was accused of taking and truly did not deserve to win the race, forfeiting the gold medal would have been a lot easier for me. But those who know me and have been with me over the past 22 years know that I took it very hard when I lost the gold medal.

Regardless of all this, today I have forgiven everyone. I hold no grudge or thoughts of revenge toward anyone. Let it be clear that I know the buck stops with me: I alone take responsibility for the lessons I came into this life to overcome.

Chaos reigned in the air and on the ground when we arrived at the airport in New York. Crowds were all over the place. Escaping media attention was impossible. Kind supporters cheered us along the way, while many just watched. The New York City Chief of Police, along with airport security and two FBI agents anxiously greeted us. They informed us there were literally hundreds of reporters and a crowd of people waiting outside for me. They advised that this could be a potentially dangerous situation for my family and me.

The FBI agents assisted us with our connecting tickets and passports and escorted us to a private room to wait for our flight. Outside through the glass windows, the media stood jostling, taking pictures but unable to speak to us. The Chief of Police and airport security stayed with us while the FBI agents went to confirm our luggage transfer and seat selection on our flight home to Toronto. When the two FBI agents came back to the room, they expressed grave disappointment. Only two seats were available on the flight to Toronto. We needed three.

My first concern was my mother and sister. I immediately suggested they go ahead without me. The agents were not comfortable with this, however. They were concerned about my safety if I were to stay in New York. They left the room again for a short time before returning with more favourable information. Miraculously, they had found one more seat on the plane.

The final leg of my journey home took place in the cockpit of the airplane. I can only imagine what the passengers in first class thought that day, watching me saunter by, escorted by FBI and airport security personnel, to the cockpit of the plane. It was the flight of my life, sitting with the pilots in the jumpseat of an American Airlines DC10.

In Toronto, a unit of airport security met us along with numerous police officers. The police were assigned to escort us through the airport to a fleet of private cars waiting outside. As I made my way through the crowd of reporters and fans, I could hear some people cheering and some crying. As if the excitement were not enough, our vehicle got a

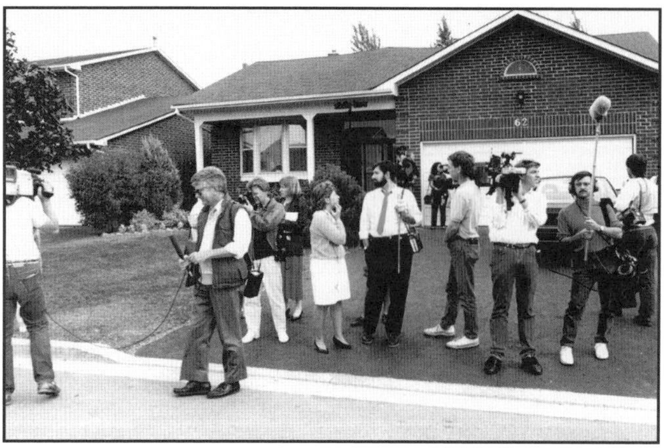

flat tire, an opportunity for the media who had been unable to get any proper photographs due to the heavy security surrounding me every step of the way. In all my life, I had never before been the target of this type of media attention. Everyone seemed to be asking the million-dollar question, "Why did you do this, Ben? Why?"

In truth, I was as bewildered as they were. Why, I wondered, too. Why did this happen to me? I absolutely knew, to the very best of my knowledge, that I had not taken stanozolol or any other steroid before my race. Moreover, everyone in my group assured me the steroid protocol we did use was completed 26 days before the competition in Seoul. This allowed more than ample time for any steroids to clear my system before the race. There was no way I should have tested positive.

The fact is steroids are widely used in sport, even though they are officially banned in the Olympics and other competitions. Like many athletes, part of my training program did include a steroid protocol. I freely admit that I did use steroids in my training. I thought they helped me to train harder and recover quicker. The theory is the steroids help as a building block for recovery by tightening the muscles after the workout. To take a steroid immediately before a race would only cause an athlete to run slower due to this muscle tightening effect. There is absolutely no advantage to taking any steroid immediately before a race. Quite the opposite, it would be a complete disadvantage. Taking steroids before a race makes no sense.

My particular steroid protocol involved cycles of usage, built around our training and competition schedules. I was always carefully supervised when using steroids. To allow the steroids to clear my system, I was very careful to make sure I stopped using them in time before a major competition. I had done this many times before. Jamie and Charlie made sure my cycle was completed weeks prior to competition. Steroids should not have been detectable in my system in Seoul. I had stopped using anything long before the required clearance time. In addition, I had been tested on August 17, 1988 at the race in Zürich. The results of these tests were negative and no banned substances were found to be in my system. Imagine, therefore, how stunned I was when they told me I tested positive after the 100 metre race in Seoul. It was just unbelievable. How could that be? Again, I can assure you, I did not knowingly do anything that would have caused me to test positive at the Seoul Olympics.

I asked Bryan to ask God, "How did my soul feel the first time I took steroids?"

Ben, you ask Me, how did your soul feel the first time you took steroids? You know the answer. The first time, you were wondering, "What is it really going to do for me? Is it going to help me run faster? Is it going to do any harm to me? Should I be doing this? Am I being given the right instructions, the right advice?" You were sitting back and thinking to yourself, saying, "I'm not an educated man. Those around me have gone through special training and I trust them." But later, hours later, your soul would start to feel indifferent, not completely supportive, questioning if you really need the steroids... because at the moment that you took the steroids, the steroids would cause you to lose confidence in your own abilities.

Bryan started to discern again. Then he looked at me and said, "The Father says that you did not tell your mother you were taking steroids until the Seoul 1988 scandal broke out. And the Father asks you, Ben, 'Do you know why you did not tell your mother before that you were taking steroids?'"

I was surprised. And I said, "This is true. I did not tell my mother I was taking steroids until 1988. I do not really know why I didn't tell her. I guess I just didn't want her to worry about me."

Bryan responded, "The Father says, this is true. This is what you believe on a conscious level. But the Father will now tell you what the Truth is, the real Truth, on a soul level:

Ben, your love for your mother is very deep. It goes back to many other soul experiences. She has always loved you deeply. She has always loved her children deeply; she wanted the best for all of her children. But most of all, she wanted her children to be honest and not to succumb to those who take advantage of the weakness of others. If you were to tell her this truth earlier, she would have done all that she could to stop you. She would have encouraged you to depend on your own abilities that I have given you. But you had a point to prove. You wanted to be able to say that you made these decisions on your own.

But I gave you your mother to guide you and to protect you. The moment you decided that day in the restaurant that you could not tell anyone, including your mother, that day with Charlie... it is that day where your protection from the Heavens was weakened because you turned your back on your mother who was the vessel for the Heavens to protect you.

But this was all written. This was all planned out. This was the story line to be. The experience of success and failure lies in taking risks, making choices. We experience the outcome and the result is always for one's soul to become wiser and to become stronger. For your soul is still on a journey, an everlasting journey, like all My Children, to learn the foundation of Truth, to learn that it is always wise to seek Truth, those of Truth, and Me in your lives.

Thank You, Father.

My mother's advice to me after Seoul was to relax, take some holidays and get some sleep. I had been training for 11 years. She said it was time to take a break, think about my future. I thought back to the days when my mom would avoid buying a new blouse, sweater or a pair of shoes, just so she could support me. She even took overtime and extra jobs to help me. She always took care of me. And now, here in my shame, she still gave me her unconditional love. She stood by me through thick and thin. She was my biggest and most loyal supporter. My dad told me outright to forget about track and field. He told me to stop running, to retire and to get an education. I told him I could not because I love to run. It was a time of real soul searching.

In the end, I received a two-year suspension from competition. I kept wondering: What happened? Why? I had trained so hard. My mother had sacrificed so much. Promises were made to my entourage. My fans were behind me. And I was a young man, not entirely familiar with business practices, following what I was told to do and doing my best to achieve what I knew I could do: win the gold medal in the men's 100 metre final. Granted, I did use steroids, but only as part of my training protocol, and definitely not before racing. I could only conclude that some sort of foul play had occurred. So, what happened?

In the bigger picture, I now accept that we are all simply actors on a stage and we are just reading our lines. I now know that my experiences with the IOC and IAAF, as well as with Carl Lewis and André Jackson, had to happen for my life to unfold the way it was written. I now understand that my life was destined to play out this way, even before I came into this life, even before I was born. Knowing this makes it much easier to forgive. I choose to forgive, rather than to walk with chronic anger or revenge. It took me 20 years to gain the ability to do this. I choose to be set free. That is the reason why only now I am able to write this book.

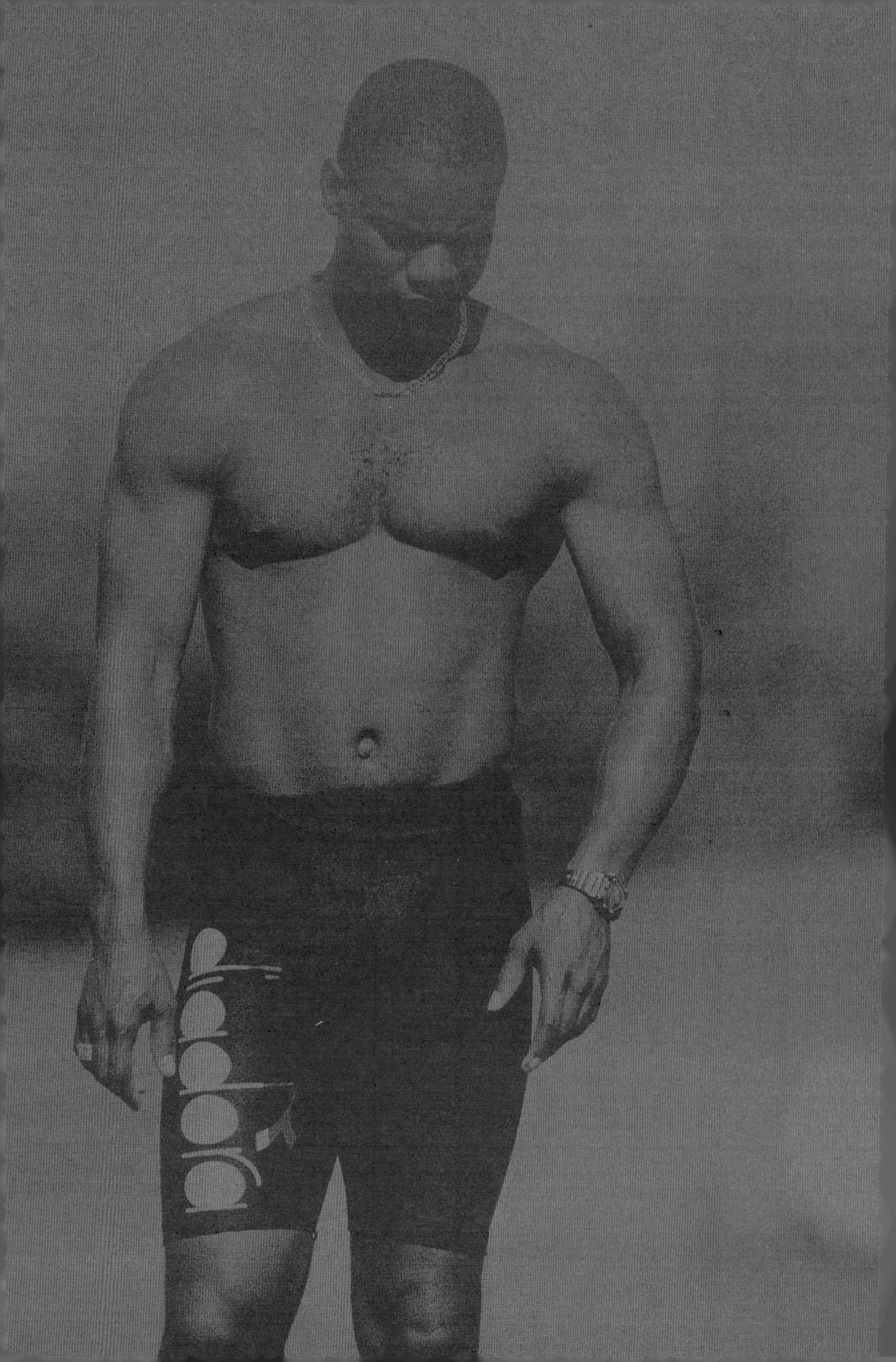

CHAPTER 3

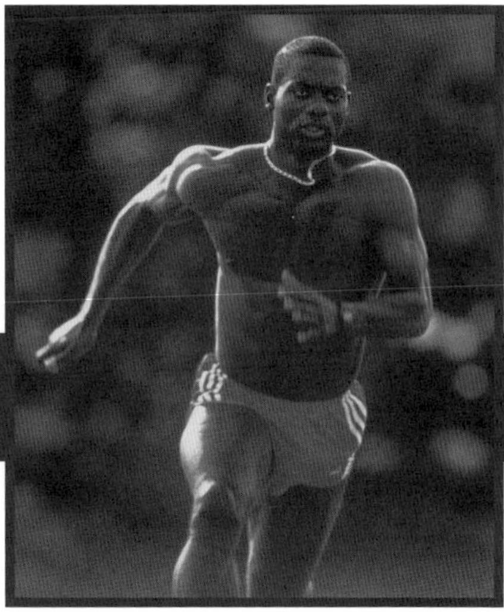

Performance-Enhancing Steroids

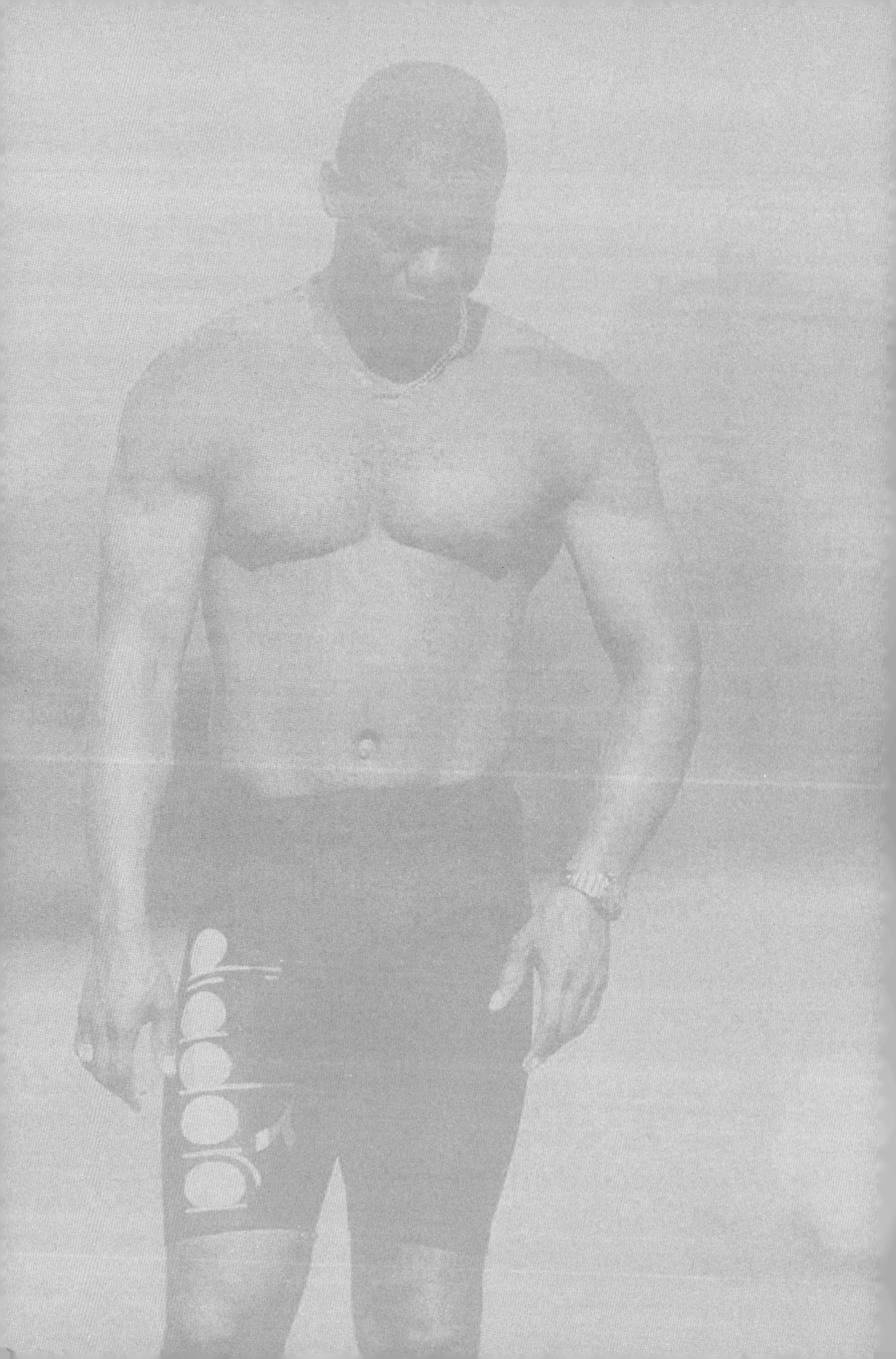

CHAPTER 3

Performance-Enhancing Steroids

As I have said before, it is true: I admit I have used steroids to help me recover after intense training. I mostly used Winstrol V, an injectable brand name of stanozolol. At one time, I used furazabol, a derivative of stanozolol. But I did not use different forms of stanozolol at the same time. I tried both at different times just to find out which one seemed to work best for me and my training regime. In addition, I also took various vitamin and mineral treatments.

Today, in 2010, this is not a shocking revelation. Since 1988, many sports figures have confirmed their own use of various performance-enhancing steroids or techniques. However, my story was one of the first, most visible, and highly publicized cases to be connected with the use of steroids in sports. Back in 1988, many athletes carefully hid any type of performance enhancement use, veiling the practice away from the glare of lights and cameras. Compared to today, few professional sports had any sort of drug testing. Those sports that did conduct testing used a process that athletes could easily circumvent.

Athletics was, still is, and probably always will be big business. The pressure to compete is intense. The mindset among many elite athletes in the 1980s was, if you did not participate in some sort of performance enhancement, you would be unfairly disadvantaged because almost every other participant did whatever was necessary to stay on top of the competition. This did not make it right. It was just the situation that existed at the time... and still does today to a certain extent.

Today, when a professional athlete like New York Yankee Alex Rodriguez tests positive, his career can continue. I thought the reason his career continued, unlike my own, was because today, there seems to be a better understanding and more willingness to forgive an athlete for these types of issues than there was in the past. I wondered about this, so I asked Bryan to discern, "Why is Alex Rodriguez still playing ball and why was he not raked over the coals like I was?"

After he discerned the Truth, Bryan responded, "Ben, throughout Alex Rodriguez's life, and even today, God plays a very strong part in his life. If you watch him, when he steps up to the plate, he will usually do the sign of the cross. This is not done for entertainment purposes. He truly believes in the power of God. When the media identified the possibility of him taking steroids, he went before God and he asked for complete forgiveness. This was granted to him."

Bryan discerned further. God spoke through him:

Ben, you remember... at the time when you lost your gold medal, throughout this experience, how many times did you come to Me and truly ask Me for help? How many times did you get down on your knees with sincerity and ask for My forgiveness? I watched you in a state of confusion, always trusting those around you. For the first time you were lost, truly lost because now you didn't know who to trust. You didn't know what to do and you just went along with the suggestions, some of which did not feel right in your heart. You got trapped into the world of the mind. The negative thoughts, at times, were overwhelming for you. All this was going on and I was waiting patiently for you to come back to Me. For the world of materialism was facing you. I ask you Ben, did any of the material experiences truly bring you joy?

I gave you your mother to be your backbone, to guide you. I gave her a spiritual gift to help protect you. I gave her the knowledge to teach you not to be so trusting, not to accept food, or drink, from a stranger. Yes, when you won the gold medal, while celebrating, you forgot about what your mother taught you.

I say to you, My son, you have not done anything wrong. These events had to take place, for the world to recognize that there is only one God. No matter what name you call Me, I Am. I shall always give My Children the option to stay with Me or to walk away from Me.

For this purpose, I have given you Bryan to help you understand why you went through the experience of winning and then losing much. But My son, you say that you have lost much, but you still have your soul. I have claim on your soul. For if a man says they have lost their soul, then, yes, they have lost much. But you, My son, you have not lost your soul. Through the remaining experience of your life, fix your heart on Me, and I will give you back much of what you believe you have lost.

Always remember: do not love anything else above or more than God; for there is nothing above Me. So to answer your question, Alex Rodriguez has always been with Me, on a deep level, that many work so hard to achieve. Alex is being used as a vessel to bring My Children back to Me. And yes, Ben, you are a vessel to bring My Children back to Me.

Two decades after the Seoul Olympics, performance-enhancing steroids are not generally accepted, but now the passage of time has revealed more to the general public about how widespread their use is. From professional athletes all the way down to the collegiate and even high school levels, the lure of being the best and the stress of competition reaches every age group and every sport.

Olympians are, and probably always will be, treated differently. The competition is even more intense: Some look forward to a life of endorsement deals and opportunities that do not come their way if they are not the winner. Second place just is not good enough, in the minds of many.

I asked Bryan, "What do I truly believe, on a soul level, about Olympic athletes?"

He said to me after discerning again, "Ben, you never believed that Olympians are professional athletes, that they are really driven for money. You believed that most athletes were driven by an eternal love for the sport, for the camaraderie with those who had a common desire to please others. Oh yes, it's true, there were some who were just in it for their own selfish motives. But most enjoy the idea of being an instrument to bring their country together, to bring hope in the eyes of the injured, to bring the world together through this one event, known as the Olympic Games. But yes, it is true, in this material world, based on its foundation of false beliefs, the act of greed and corruption has penetrated the sport and has poisoned the hearts of many."

The first time I ever heard of athletes using steroids was in the early 1980s. As time went on, it became common knowledge among track and field insiders that the practice had become widespread. But I had never personally participated in its use until Charlie Francis made the proposal to me in the early eighties.

I asked Bryan to discern, to ask God, "How did I truly feel, on a soul level, when Charlie Francis first presented the option to me to take steroids?"

Ben, going back to the first time that you took steroids, you were not sure about steroids. You trusted those around you. But you did not trust in yourself... you failed to believe truly, at that time, that sprinters are born, they are not made.

I gave you the genetics to be a sprinter. For so many, through their own jealousy, had a very difficult time accepting that you were given this gift while they wished, prior to coming into this life, that they would have the same gift. There is a Math Equation of God that all of My Children are part of, and this time around, that Math Equation allowed you to have the genetics of being born as a sprinter.

For those who gave you the steroids, gave you the steroids to change the mirror that they had been looking at. For their own mirror showed that they had anger of not being born the sprinter. For each time they watched you race, they watched you win, their anger grew. Steroids are one way to remove the mirror that reflected the anger that they hold within.

When I heard this Truth, I said, "When it's all said and done, I forgive all."

Charlie presented the steroid injections to me as special vitamins, explaining that most, if not all, of the top competitors were using some type of performance-enhancement. He told me, if I wished to compete on the same playing field with the big boys, I had to use them, too. The theory was: it would level the playing field and even the odds. Moreover, Jamie Astaphan and Charlie both claimed it was best to submit to a formal program that would be professionally supervised, rather than to rely on novices or on my own application. I went along with the steroid protocol suggestions of Charlie and Jamie because of my fear that if I had refused, they would not back me and continue to train me. I trusted they would look out for my best interests. I chose to believe them and I chose to simply leave all the details to the professionals.

Looking back today, I often wonder whether corporate greed to sell athletic shoes serves, on some level, to encourage athletes to take steroids, based on promises of big payouts through sponsorship deals. Was it my own personal greed that ultimately caused me to fail? The answer is yes.

If I had a chance to do it again, based on my experiences, I would choose not to take steroids at all. Furthermore, I would encourage others not to succumb to the pressure and avoid steroid use or any other performance-enhancing applications completely. I asked Bryan to ask God why, on a deeper level, I took the steroids in the first place.

Ben, you ask why you took steroids in the first place. I say to you: Why does someone smoke cigarettes? Why does someone bring harm against themselves? Why do My Children punish themselves? Ben, on some level, you felt abandoned. You felt rejected. The closeness of your father, your biological father, your earthly father, was not there completely for you. Your father was a wise man. Did I not give him wisdom? If your father was to truly nourish you with love, would you have been so determined to go all the way? Would you have stopped half way? Would you have given up? There is a deeper reason why you were determined to be a track star: For if the world would accept you, you believed your father, your earthly father, would have accepted you. The appreciation, the acknowledgment was not always there. His love was not always there. For it was not written for him to love you the way that you believed you needed to be loved. The separation between you and your earthly father made you stronger and made you more determined.

But I say to you, Ben, because your father rejected you emotionally, at some point in your life, in your childhood, you felt unworthy. You also came into this world with memories of other incarnations that caused you to feel unworthy, not deserving. This soul memory that you brought into this world was like a cement block around your ankles. The only way this block was able to be lifted was to come back to Me. I have lifted this block from you. I have lifted the pain from you. And I have lifted many of your false beliefs from you. From this moment on, trust only in Me.

I looked down, shook my head a bit, sighed, and I said it was true. I was always trying to fill my father's shoes.

In the Olympics and other high-profile international sporting events, it is not just the athletes who compete. The countries compete as well. On such a large public stage, another layer of expectation exists from a political standpoint: No country wants to be humiliated. I have been accused of tarnishing Canadian sports and embarrassing the Canadian public. Since my experience in Seoul, many others have admitted using some sort of performance enhancement. But I took the brunt of the heat.

Maybe it was because of the spectacular nature of my achievement. Or, perhaps it was because I was the most famous Canadian at that point in time. I could not help but think if I had been on the American team, this would never have been allowed to happen. Rather than supporting athletes, delving deeper and finding solutions, as the Americans can do, the Canadian reaction was simply to reject me. As some reminded me after Seoul, I was born in Jamaica, after all.

I wanted to ask Bryan to ask God about this, because it still really bothered me. I asked, "Did Canada actually reject me?"

Ben, for you ask the question, did the people of Canada truly reject you as a result of you losing your gold medal? You must understand: Canada did not reject you. They rejected how you were treated unfairly. This is the disappointment that many Canadians have. They do not have all the facts. They do not know what happened to you and what you did, and how this knowledge impacted your life. This life, all was set in stone before you came into your mother's womb. For all who participated in you losing the gold medal had specific roles to allow you to get to this point: to teach My Children the importance of forgiveness. But you must always remember: the people of your country, that you live in, have been good to you. They only rejected the unfairness of many toward you. And as this was going on, their hands were tied. At this time in your life, the rope around your hands and around the hands of Canadians is about to be cut.

Don't you know this is true? When you walk down the street, don't most Canadians come up to you and say, "Ben, I know you were cheated," or, "I know you were treated unfairly," or they say, "I'm proud of you." Ben, is this not true? So I say to you, how can the people of Canada reject you?

I smiled in agreement with the statement. This does happen to me a lot, people approaching with kind words. It even happened to me the very morning that I received this discernment. After Seoul, I admit I was disappointed with the way the media attacked me. Understandably though, like myself at the time, the media did not know how I was sabotaged and by whom. No one knew the truth.

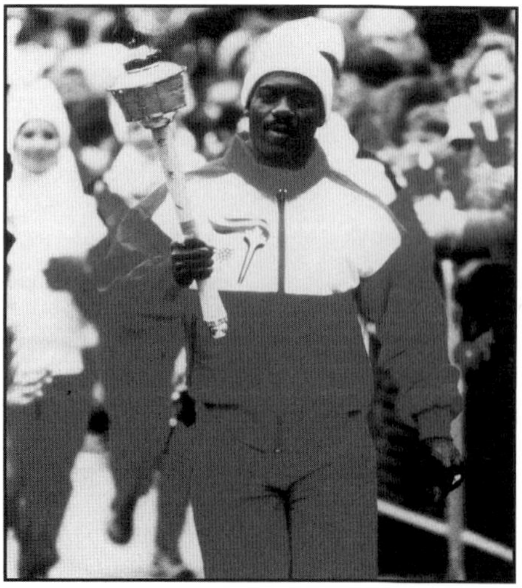

Overnight, I became the notorious poster boy for steroid abuse in sports. I carried the flag for Canada at the opening ceremonies of the Commonwealth Games in Edinburgh, Scotland in 1986 and was proud to do so. I carried the Olympic torch into Toronto before the Seoul games in 1988. But ever since Seoul, I have carried the mark of "disgraced sprinter, Ben Johnson."

I asked Bryan, "Why did I come into this life to be the disgraced poster boy for steroids?" God answered:

Ben, as I speak these words to you, as these words are printed, for many will not understand or even accept this Truth. There is not one human being on this planet, on a soul level, that truly believes you were treated fairly at the Seoul Olympics. And they do not believe you actually cheated. It is just like there is not one human being on this planet, on a soul level, who truly believes that Christ was of the dark. So you may ask

Me, "How is this possible?" I say to you and to all My Children of the world: there is only One Soul in the universe and My Children share a fragment of that One Soul. So the Truth in the One Soul says that you did not cheat in Seoul, that you were treated unfairly. So, since all My Children share the One Soul, they all share the same Truth.

He paused and went on:

Ben, those who continue to judge you, actually judge themselves. For you become the mirror reflection for those who have not forgiven themselves for what they have done unto others. For many simply wish that the name, Ben Johnson... Ben Johnson... Ben Johnson... simply goes away, as the mirror that they look into is too intense for them. There are others who look at the mirror and wish so desperately they could have had a similar experience of becoming recognized as a gold medalist. Because they did not achieve this, they have become extremely jealous. On some level, on some recount of another soul experience, they may have failed in a similar way. But in every case, those who judge others never wish to see another happy. For those same individuals to see you happy, Ben, to see you reclaim your name becomes a huge threat to them as they revisit the mirror once again. It is easier for them to try to crack, smash, destroy the mirror because they fear revisiting that mirror.

Even 22 years after Seoul, the veil of secrecy surrounding performance enhancement use was so well-woven that the general public still does not know the full extent of how deeply rooted the problem was, and continues to be, in almost every area of sport. Approximately 82 international athletes have been tested and identified as users of banned substances during the Olympic Games held between 1972 in Munich and 2004 in Athens. Seven athletes tested positive in Munich, ten in Montréal, twelve in LA, nine in Seoul. This may come as a surprise since many people assume I was the only one who tested positive in Seoul. Five were discovered in 1992 in Barcelona, two in Atlanta, ten in Sydney and a whopping 27 in Athens.

Some would say this is proof that the anti-doping system is working. Testing has become more sensitive. However, testing is not addressing the core root of the problem: the mindset that an athlete must use performance enhancement to be competitive. From my own experience and what I have seen while competing, these disclosures are a mere tip of the iceberg. The culture of "use but don't get caught" continues in many sports and at many Olympic events. I asked Bryan to shed some light on the mindset of athletes that take steroids.

Bryan discerned for a minute and then said, "Ben, on a soul level, athletes do not take steroids to become more competitive. They take steroids to punish themselves. And this is what the world needs to know. This is why it is important for counseling and spirituality to have a dominant influence in the Olympics: to help the athletes heal their own personal issues of unworthiness. Once these issues have been removed, the athlete would have no desire to take steroids.

"Now, many will disagree with me. And many will not believe that God speaks through me. But even for the scientists, they speak so wonderfully about the atom when they have not even seen the atom. They speak of electricity and yet, they cannot tell you how electricity works. They speak of the human cell and their knowledge is not more than 5% of the complete Truth about the cell. And yet, they make life-challenging decisions based only on this 5%. For they use the word, theory. But when they are asked directly, 'Do you actually believe this theory is truth? Complete truth?' very few can answer yes."

Then God began to address me:

But they say that I do not exist. They are disconnected from their soul and it is their own spirit that continually confuses them. I say to you, the human spirit, on some level, represents separation from God and the soul represents connection to God. Those who know Me, know Me through their soul; those who do not know Me are held hostage by their own spirit, by their own false beliefs.

Of the 82 international athletes who tested positive during the eight games mentioned above, it is interesting to note that only five were from the USA. That's right, only five Americans! One swimmer in Munich. Two weightlifters in Montréal. Two in Barcelona. And that's it. Zero in LA. Zero in Seoul. Zero in Atlanta. Zero in Sydney. And zero in Athens. What does this say? Does it mean that the US athletes, or any other countries' athletes, are free of performance enhancement? We know from recent admissions of current and past Olympians that they are not: they just did not get caught.

I asked Bryan why other Olympic athletes who took steroids around the time of Seoul did not test positive. Bryan discerned and then replied, "Yes, Ben. Some of the athletes, through their special relationships, were protected. This is true. But that is not important. What's important is for all to realize that steroids do more harm than good."

Six out of the eight sprinters that lined up to compete against me in Seoul have since been exposed for performance enhancement before or after the Seoul Olympics. I am hopeful that Carl Lewis will tell his story one day, the real and true story of how he dealt with the pressure and navigated the existing drug rule. He has always had a story, and he is not someone who would allow an opportunity to pass without having something to say.

After the 1987 World Championships in Rome, Carl explained his loss by pointing fingers. He insisted that there were gold medalists who were definitely on drugs. It was clear to everyone that he was referring to me. The media, of course, took his words seriously. Immediately, I was forced to answer to the allegation. My response was simple: When Carl Lewis was winning I never said a word against him publicly. He won and that was it. We both knew what was going on behind the scenes and that this was a dangerous and double-edged accusation he had made.

Ironically, Carl almost did not compete in Seoul. In 2003, Sports Illustrated exposed a report they had received from a former high-ranking US Olympic official. This report had a list of some 100 US athletes who had failed their drug tests, but who were still allowed to compete. Carl Lewis's name was on that list. According to the report, Carl tested positive three times before the 1988 Olympic Games for having banned stimulants in his system. He was subsequently banned from competing in Seoul three weeks before the competition. Others from his Santa Monica track club were also on the list. Carl and his team, however, appealed the decision, saying that use of the substance was inadvertent. The United States Olympic Committee then reversed their decision and allowed Carl to compete in Seoul.

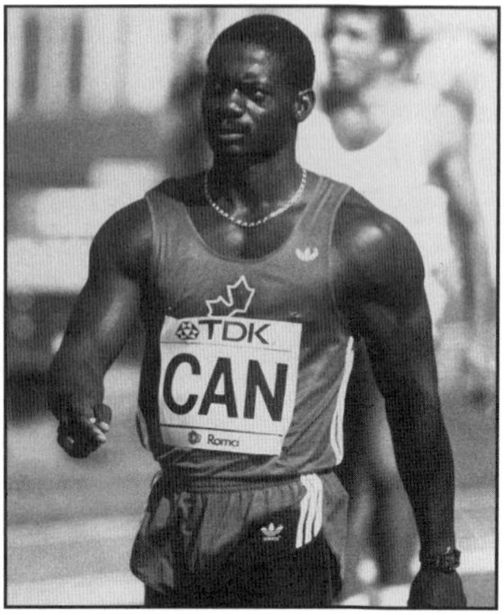

I was afraid not to take the advice of my doctor, my coach and others who told me taking steroids was a necessary step I needed to be able to train with the level of intensity that was required. My training regimen placed a heavy demand on my body. Because of performance-enhancing substances, I believed I was able to train longer, recover quicker, and sustain my training for short-term intervals. When I took steroids, I realized that it would allow me to be pain-free six hours after training. Then if I did not take steroids the next day, my body, my muscle tissue would ache for up to four days afterward, impairing my athletic capability. While I was on steroids, I had to be careful I did not get dehydrated: I noticed that I became less thirsty. I drank less water. I also noticed that I had many restless nights when I was taking steroids.

I asked Bryan, "What did steroids really do to my body?" God answered my question:

Ben, the use of steroids did not help you win any races. In fact, when you did use steroids, it slowed you down. For one to be free of the short-term negative impact of steroids, one must be free of steroids anywhere from 90 to 120 days. The steroids are there to create an electrical imbalance in the body that can cripple different cells from communicating with each other. The steroids are able to create a hormonal imbalance in the body that can cause premature bone aging. The steroids used over a long period of time can cause an impairment of one's short-term memory and cause an impairment of one's ability to think logically. Steroids can alter one's state of reality, where common sense simply becomes a fantasy. Steroids over time decrease the ability to focus and to be able to be directionally competent, meaning intelligence capabilities at times may be compromised. Steroids can impact up to 11 different organs in the body, the communication between organs being directed from the heart. The steroids, over time, can weaken the heart wall and can thicken the arteries. Steroids place much stress on the liver and it can compromise up to 24 different stem cells. As well, steroids may cause the soul to be separated from the heart, causing a loss of intuitive ability, which causes further dependence on the mind instead of the heart. Always remember: Our soul is always a friend to us. Our mind can often play tricks on us.

Steroids do not help sprinters win races. The steroids simply give another a need, a purpose: to look after the athlete who has been taking the steroids. So the benefit for one to take the steroids is not with the athlete; but instead, it is with those individuals who create their life purpose around the athlete.

In hindsight, I only wish I had loved myself more. I only wish I had a closer, more loving relationship with my father, whom I loved very much. And I wish I had not come into this life with soul baggage that caused me to feel unworthy and punish myself by taking the steroids. Many would believe the price I paid was in money lost. But I know the real cost to me was embarrassment and humiliation, having my dream taken away from me, recognizing clearly I must take complete self-accountability and responsibility for all that happened.

I asked Bryan to discern whether or not taking steroids actually improves anybody's performance. God responded to my question:

Ben, for many ask this question. Is there a benefit, a true benefit, in performance if one should take steroids? There are many other questions that still need to be asked and answered in connection to steroids. Back in Seoul in 1988, the general knowledge of steroid use, and its impact on performance and on the body, the physical body, was inadequate. Does one drug have the same impact on everyone? Do all drugs truly work? Is it the drug or the impact of belief empowering the mind to cause another chemical response in the body? For if one takes steroids and truly believes there is no benefit, can that steroid increase their performance? If one takes steroids and believes that the steroids can improve their performance, will their performance increase?

Steroids in almost every case act as a placebo. Is it not simply the mind believing that the steroid is giving them more advantage, more power, more strength? Again, is this not a placebo, if one believes?

For My Children must understand: In science today, much that is presented to the world does not have a strong foundation. For anything that is less than Truth in science is known as theory. If the science of steroids was correctly understood at the time that you lost your gold medal, steroids would not have been an issue, you would not have lost your gold medal and the Dubin Inquiry would not have taken place.

I am hoping this book will provide better understanding of what happened to me, as well as bring to light many issues surrounding circumstances of that day in Seoul. I was unfairly made the scapegoat: I became the example for all other steroid users. As far as some people are concerned, this is my only legacy.

I asked Bryan to discern, "What is my spiritual legacy?" Bryan closed his eyes again to discern. The fingers of his right hand moved as though he was flipping through my spiritual file, held in God's Archives in the Heavens.

Bryan opened his eyes and said, "Ben, you seek to understand your spiritual legacy. For your legacy is very simple to say, but very difficult to understand. You shall be remembered as the example of what happens when one has not included God in one's life. And you shall be remembered afterward as the example of what happens to one who claims God back into one's life. For you are the example. For this is your legacy."

The only way I survived the 22 years after Seoul was through inner strength, holding on to my faith and the love and support of my family. I have sincerely forgiven all who have harmed me. In my heart, I truly know I am on my way to being set free.

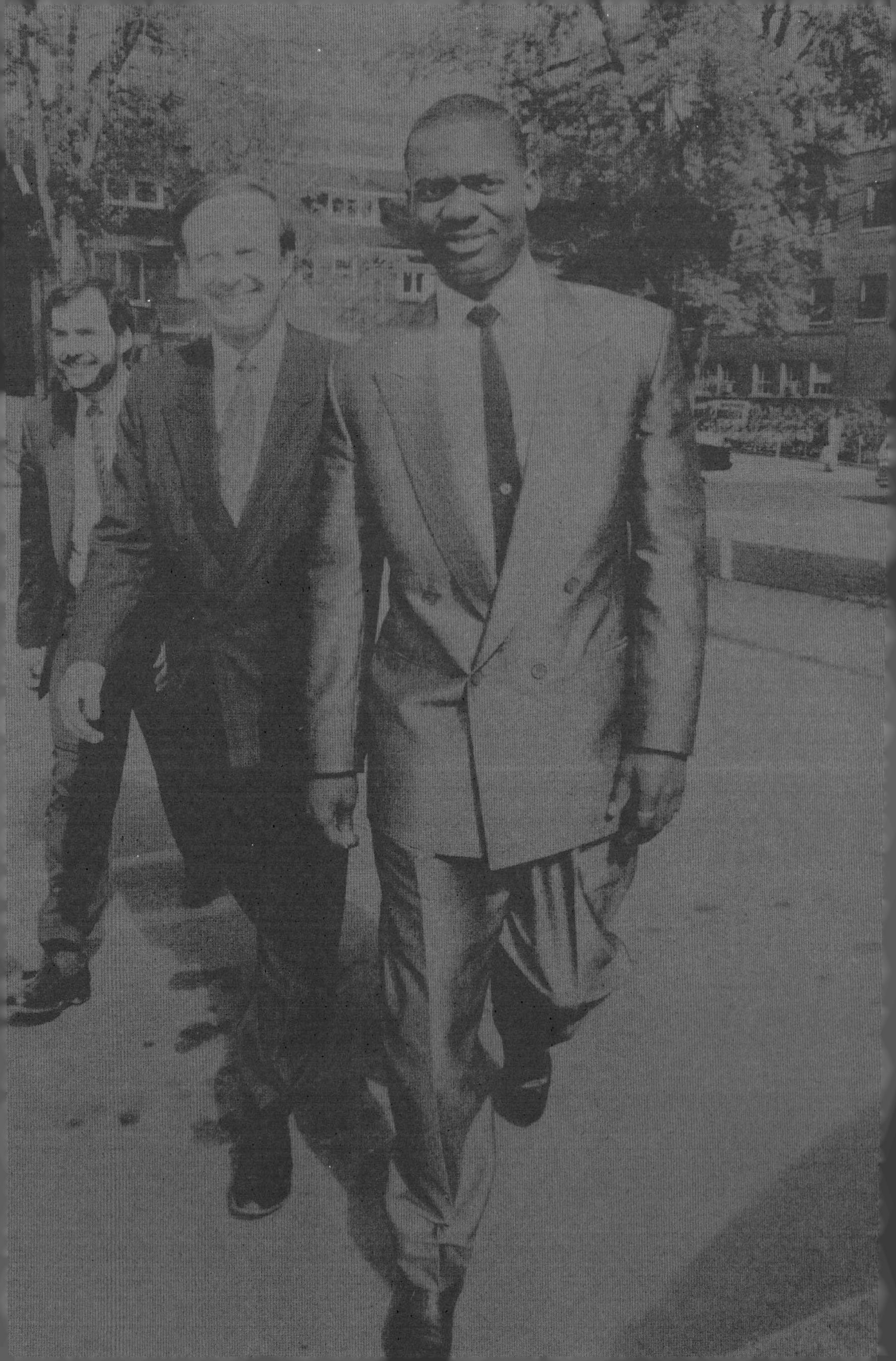

CHAPTER 4

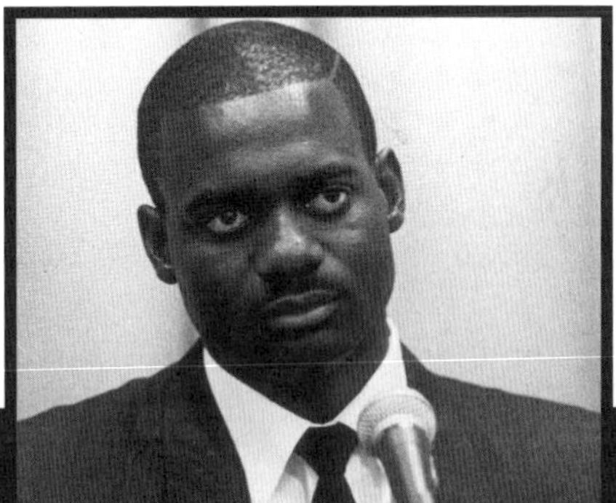

The Dubin Inquiry

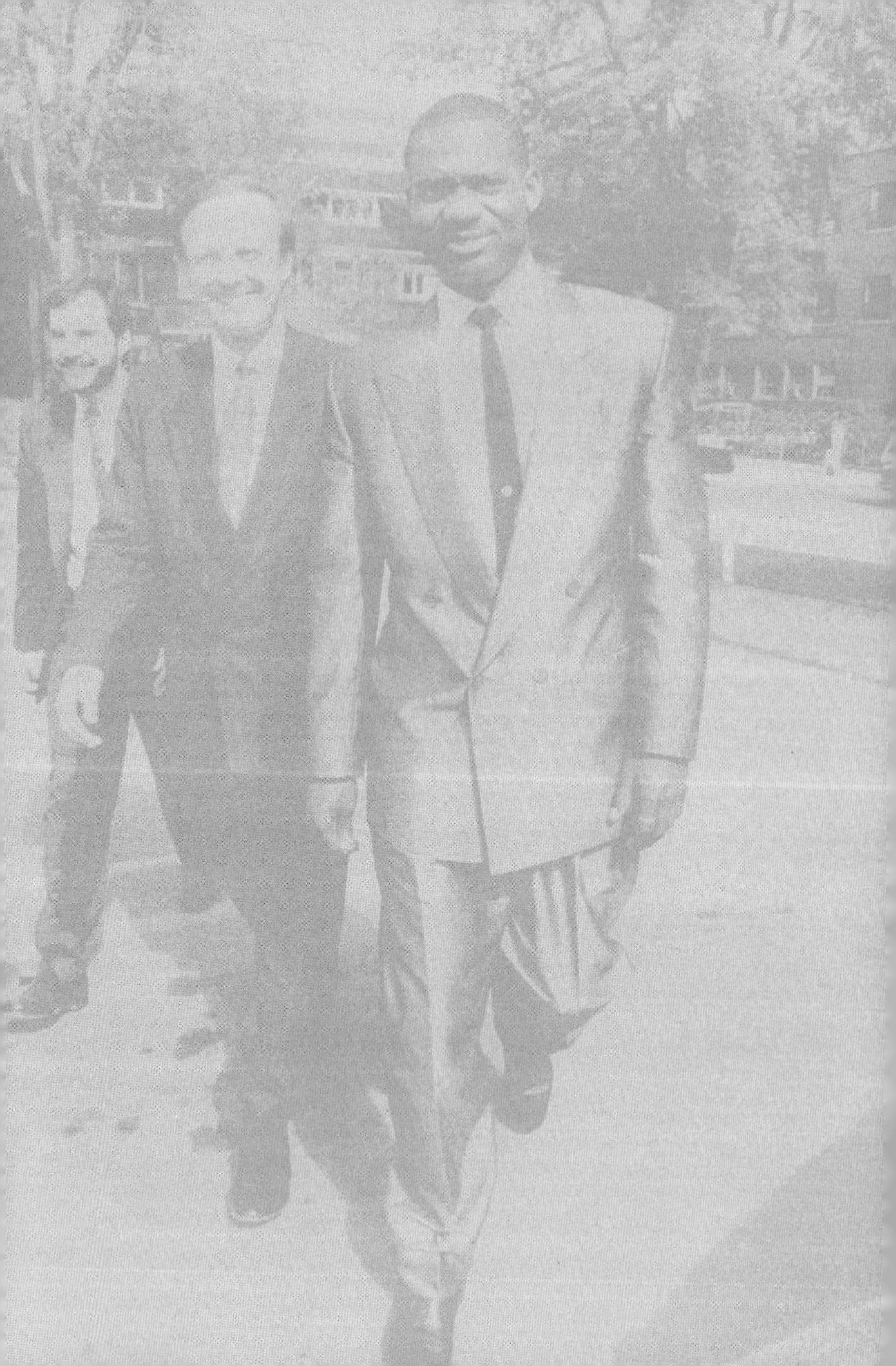

CHAPTER 4

The Dubin Inquiry

After the positive steroid test in Seoul, the authorities not only stripped me of my gold medal, they also suspended me from competition for two years. In addition, the two world records I set in Seoul and in Rome were declared null and void. They were wiped from the record books.

I was 27 years old. I had passed up my education and had been running for more than a third of my life. Here I was, facing a complicated situation I had never faced before, one that was being played out on the world stage. I have to admit it was a very confusing time for me. To those around me, I guess it seemed like I needed all the help I could get. And I did, but many took advantage of my time of need and my trusting nature. Many people approached me to offer their help and advice. Some were genuine and sincere. But there were also others who were only looking out for themselves. People around me were under a great deal of pressure trying to defend themselves and protect their own perceived integrity.

Today, I understand these circumstances better. The people who were supposed to protect me were not able to completely do so. They were unable to protect my integrity because, at that time, the complete truth was not available. No one knew that André Jackson had spiked my beer. This vital information had not yet been made available to everyone. If André had come forward to confess at that point, my name would have been cleared. But obviously, this was not meant to be.

When I was five months into my suspension, the Dubin Inquiry began. Prime Minister Mulroney appointed Ontario's Associate Chief Justice Charles Dubin to head the Inquiry. Mr. Justice Dubin was the sole commissioner and the Inquiry became named after him.

My advisors believed the Inquiry was going to help me. I agreed with them. I thought if everyone looked at the situation honestly and thoroughly investigated and reviewed all the facts, they would conclude that I was sabotaged. Furthermore, they would see that corruption existed in the sport and the use of steroids was not restricted to just me or even only a handful of athletes. I naïvely thought this was what it would take for Canada to realize how unfairly I had been treated. I honestly believed the Inquiry would uncover the truth and help me figure out exactly how I was sabotaged in Seoul.

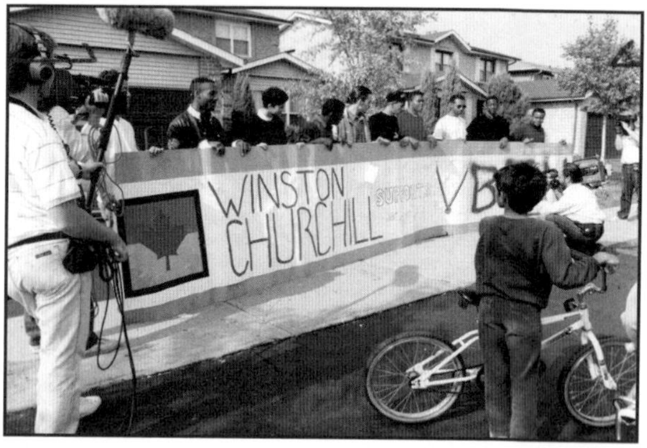

The official mandate of the Inquiry was to look into the use of steroids and banned substances in sports. The Sports Minister at the time, Jean Charest, proclaimed the purpose of the Inquiry: to restore the integrity of sport in Canada. I asked Bryan to ask God about Jean Charest's intent.

Ben, you asked me about Jean Charest. Did he have a pure intent in supporting the Dubin Inquiry? I will confirm to you he did have a pure intent. He was very disappointed that you lost the gold medal, as were many other Canadians, as were many other people in countries around the world. It was a huge shock for many who followed your career. Mr. Charest is not a man of prejudice against different ethnicities or races. He was hoping that, through this Inquiry, your name would be cleared... just like many Canadians, many around the world and, yes, even many in the media were hoping your name would be cleared.

I only wish I knew at the time of this Inquiry how the sabotage of my doping test had taken place.

During the Inquiry, I found it very difficult to stay positive. I knew I was innocent, but back then I did not have the knowledge and spiritual wisdom that would have enabled me to clear my name. This was an extremely challenging time for me, having my personal life exposed to the world yet not getting the support I needed to clear my name. I did not know for certain what truly had happened to me in Seoul and exactly how it had taken place. I did not have the truth that I know today, the truth about how I was sabotaged by André Jackson.

My uncertainty and underlying emotional pain made it very difficult for me to communicate effectively. My speech impairment only compounded the problem. It was hard for people to comprehend me and it was hard for everyone involved to understand what the truth was.

I tried to remain as calm as possible. I knew it would not have done any good to fall apart now after all I had already been through. I had to just get through this somehow, hoping and praying I could remain healthy enough to run again after my two-year suspension. Seoul was like a catastrophic earthquake and the Dubin Inquiry was just one of the many tremors afterward that I had to face.

At every turn, there were rumours being spread about my use of and attitude toward steroids. Some claimed that steroids were all I talked about, that I would routinely give steroids to others. While these statements were damaging my reputation further, I knew they were not true. But my hands were tied.

I simply did not know how to address the media. I knew reporters needed to have answers. But I was very frustrated because, again, I did not know exactly what the truth was. I could not give an intelligent response. I was unable to answer the tough questions I was asked. Some members of the press falsely accused me of giving steroids to others. This was most definitely not the case. It was very difficult for me to deal with these false statements. But I understand now the journalists were only doing their job, trying to get the truth out.

I asked Bryan to discern the Truth about the media. I wanted to know why many reporters treated me in what seemed an unfair manner. Bryan discerned that there is much competition among the media to obtain news stories and report the facts correctly. Some journalists have a desire to become very popular, to become the most trusted reporter at the expense of another, not really caring about reporting truth but instead, only caring about creating sensationalism.

I am not judging the press. I am not criticizing the press. I am only expressing how I felt and what I went through, the mix of various emotions from becoming trapped in a cocoon of misinformation. I was not able to get out of that cocoon because, once again, I did not know André Jackson had spiked my beer. I certainly wish I had obtained that information during the Inquiry. I wish I could have given that information to the press. If I had, I know they would have acted differently toward me.

Today, I have forgiven those individuals in the press who accused me falsely. I have no resentment toward the media. I am on a spiritual path, striving to cleanse my soul on an ongoing basis. I know that life is not always easy. I know that my own personal weakness in trusting people too much has been a challenge for me and for others. Today, I am not as trusting. And I have become much more selective about whom I choose to include as part of my spiritual path. I will continue to learn the lessons this spiritual path provides, whatever those lessons are. One day, I hope to be able to look at another and only find love reflected back to me in everyone I see.

All along I maintained that I did not win in Seoul because I took steroids. I won because of my God-given talent: I was the fastest, plain and simple. I asked Bryan to ask God, "Why did I win in Seoul?"

Ben, you ask the question, why did you win the 100m race? You believe it is your own ability that caused you to win. This is partly true. It is not true that you won because of steroid use. It is true that there was something else that drove you to run faster... that drove you from your kidneys... that drove you from your adrenal glands... that drove you from your pituitary gland... that drove you from your basal ganglia... that drove you from your testosterone. For what is it that helped to create the chemical response in your physical body to cause you to run so quickly?

My child, fear can cause one to do great things. Fear can cause a mother to lift a car with incredible strength in order for her child to be pulled out from underneath. This is the same fear that drove you to win the race... that gave you that extra strength... that created the chemical response for you to achieve the objective. For you were well focused. I made you this way. It was your fear of not being number one... your fear of not pleasing many... because it is your desire to please others, even above yourself. Even as you were rewarded with much of the material world throughout your career, it never sat well with you. This is not how I made you. For you are one to please others. You are one to please Me.

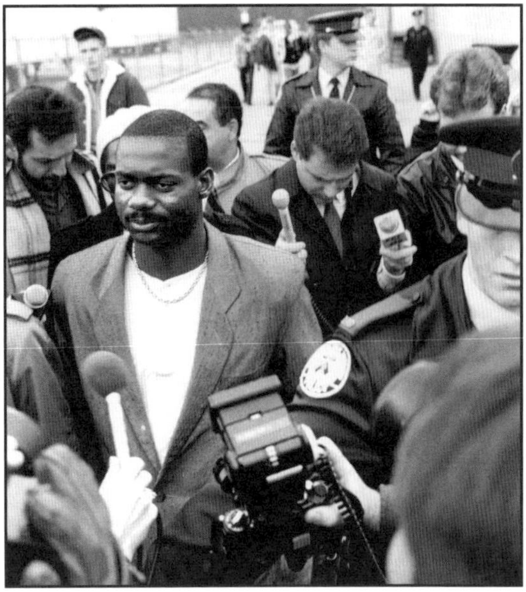

I sat back, taking all this in. I reflected back over my life and my running career and I knew everything God said to me through Bryan was true. Thinking back to my time in Seoul, I remember the fear I felt within. The dominant thought driving me was, "I'm not going to lose this race: Victory will be mine." That was my destiny and that is what I trained to do throughout my racing career.

When my mother was alive, she often gave me good advice. She told me to speak the truth at all cost. And that is what I did when it was my turn to actually speak for myself at the Dubin Inquiry. My father also believed in me and knew this mess was bigger than just me. After 92 days, I was the last of 122 witnesses to be called before the commission. Experts, coaches, administrators, government officials, and doctors had gone before me to testify. Charlie and my teammates also testified. When my turn came, there was really nothing left for me to add, except to admit to prior use of steroids and to apologize publicly. My hands were tied because, again, I did not have the complete truth about how I was sabotaged.

Unbeknownst to the public, before the Dubin Inquiry, my lawyer arranged for me to take a lie detector test in Boston. I was asked many questions at the time of the test. Afterward, I was told I had passed the test. But this did not matter. The evidence was not admissible at the Dubin Inquiry under Canadian legal statutes.

I asked Bryan to discern why the lie detector test I took was not used as evidence in the Dubin Inquiry. God answered:

Ben, you ask the question, why was the lie detector test that you took not used as evidence in the Dubin Inquiry? My son, for many ask the question, "Why did Simon Peter denounce Christ three times?" Many around you had fear of speaking the Truth. They protected themselves. Some were afraid of the consequences. What is a lie detector test? For is this Truth? Is this Truth in every case? The chemical brain structures, the physical body's chemical reactions, can cause the spoken word to appear as truth when it is not truth... a lie.

The journey for you has been written. The higher purpose for the experience that you went through is for you to act as a vessel by written word, by your biography. For many who are turning away from their church today can be easily influenced by those who pretend to know Me. For your life is to be an instrument for many to return back to Me. For the story must evolve, as it is written to be completed, so that you and My Children will have an understanding that there is a God, a very forgiving God, a very loving God, a God Who does not punish.

I am really going to need God's help because I cannot do it alone.

At the end of the Inquiry, I think Mr. Justice Dubin understood steroid use in the sport was more widespread than anyone first believed. I think he also realized the possibility of large financial gain motivated some athletes' extreme need to win. He disagreed with the IAAF's decision to retroactively strip me of my previous record and called into question the Canadian sports body for some of its rules and policies. He admitted he doubted future records likely to replace mine would be steroid-free.

I asked Bryan to ask God about Mr. Justice Dubin.

Ben, you ask me about Mr. Justice Dubin. For his role was written for him. Even though it appeared that he did not treat you well, I say unto you: his role, in the end, will turn out to help you much more than you can ever imagine. For I know you have forgiven this man. And his response to you was always in accordance with what was written in his spiritual contract that needed to be fulfilled to get you to the point where you are today.

I said in reply, "Well, that's great. I really do not wish to have the same Dubin Inquiry experience again."

And Bryan responded, "Yes, I understand, Ben. But through time, you will find that Justice Charles Dubin really did help you in a big way. And remember Ben, as long as you are free of anger toward Justice Charles Dubin, or toward anyone, you cannot have the spirit of revenge toward another."

I have forgiven all.

I was encouraged by Mr. Justice Dubin's words. Clearly, he saw part of the bigger picture. Nevertheless, the Inquiry failed to vindicate me personally. Even after learning of the politics of the IOC, COA and IAAF, not to mention the huge financial profits to be gained, Mr. Justice Dubin still did not consider the possibility that I had been sabotaged in Seoul. There was no acknowledgement, investigation or consideration that my urine sample could have been interfered with, or that others could have conspired to set me up. No investigation of André Jackson or the legitimacy of a mystery man's presence in the doping area ever took place.

For me, at the time, this was a major breakdown in the process of due diligence. No one would even consider my assertion that André should not have had access to me in the doping room. They even went so far as to claim no one could possibly have been in the room with me.

However, in 1990, Carl Lewis published two photographs in his book, Inside Track. These photographs clearly prove André was in the testing waiting room with me. One photo even shows the beer cans on the floor. These photos have been a constant reminder to me of the possibility that maybe Carl could have been involved. I would like to see André Jackson, or anyone else who was in the room that day with me, take a lie detector test, as I have done. Even though I have forgiven André, in man's world people will still require man's proof that I'm speaking the truth. If it wasn't for this need for substantiation, I would not care one way or another whether André Jackson decided to take the lie detector test or not. Even if Carl Lewis wants to take a lie detector test, I do not care one way or another. I know in my heart that I have made peace with myself. I have made peace with God.

The Inquiry also neglected to investigate the finding of Professor Arnold Beckett. Professor Beckett, who has very recently passed away, had told me in Seoul that the amount of stanozolol found in my urine was enough to be a lethal dose. Again, this was yet another fact that should have warranted a full investigation into the possibility of tampering. But admitting evidence of tampering would have opened the door to officials acknowledging security was breached in the doping area and those in charge had failed to protect me. I can only conclude this is partly the reason my test results were not scrutinized in a much more attentive manner.

In addition, the Inquiry failed to probe into the complex relationship of sponsors, broadcasting rights, money and profit, and how they are linked with athletic performance. If the Dubin Inquiry had scrutinized this link, it could have revealed that the over-arching problem was not just the athletes themselves, but also the corporate giants who make their millions marketing sports icons. I believe that the sabotage of my race was an elaborate scheme involving many players, the success of which secured certain multi-million-dollar contracts and endorsements for Carl Lewis. The IOC testing is one way to manipulate the outcome of the Games from behind the scenes. But Members of the IOC should not be taking part in any activity with respect to sponsorships for athletes since this is a clear conflict of interest.

There was, and still is, intense pressure placed on athletes. I don't think Mr. Justice Dubin fully understood or appreciated that. Had the Inquiry gone differently, it could have been about more than just me. It could have extended beyond a simple steroid scandal. It could have been about money and greed corrupting the purity of sport. It could have called André Jackson, Carl Lewis, his coach Joe Douglas and others to testify.

I was not the first athlete caught in the web of corporate power and I will not be the last. As elite athletes, we court the support, financial success and security that endorsements can bring. But we also run the risk of becoming corrupted in order to keep those endorsements.

On a political level, Canadian-US relations were at a very sensitive point as they were negotiating the North American Free Trade Agreement (NAFTA) during the time period of the Dubin Inquiry. Someone once suggested to me that I had been used as a pawn in these sensitive negotiations to keep the US content. I asked Bryan to discern if this was truly the case.

God gave me the Truth:

Ben, again you ask another question, as you wish to know if you truly were a pawn, if your name, Ben Johnson, was on the political table among American and Canadian government officials. You must go back into your childhood and remember the uncertainties that you experienced... the uncertainty of not knowing, of not understanding.

Is it not true that you would like to do things your way? And when you do not have your way, you try to interpret what is going on, asking the question to yourself, why? But you did not always ask the question why. You did not always take the time to understand. In many cases, you went with the first impression, which was not always the Truth. In sports, throughout school, you would try to do it your way. And at times, it worked out. And other times, it did not... thinking that maybe someone else was responsible, and not always looking within yourself, not trying to understand the limitations that you may have. For when I created you, yes, you were created to trust someone 100% until they have proven to you they no longer can be trusted.

Some of the information that you may have received around the time of Seoul, with respect to your name being on the table, was not completely correct. One way or another, it would have made no difference in the outcome of the trade deal. Focus on going within and looking for the answer within. Everybody had a role to play, even the governments of Canada and the United States, for they have helped you much. Many have helped you greatly. Now you have great inner spiritual strength. You have become wiser and you have learned not to trust so much in man, but to trust in your inner intuition. Listen to your body, for that's where you will know the

Truth, for you will feel the Truth in your heart and if it is not truthful, you will feel uneasiness in your stomach. For this is what you must go with from this moment on. Trust only in Me.

I wish my mother were alive to have the experience of meeting Bryan. She would have been overjoyed.

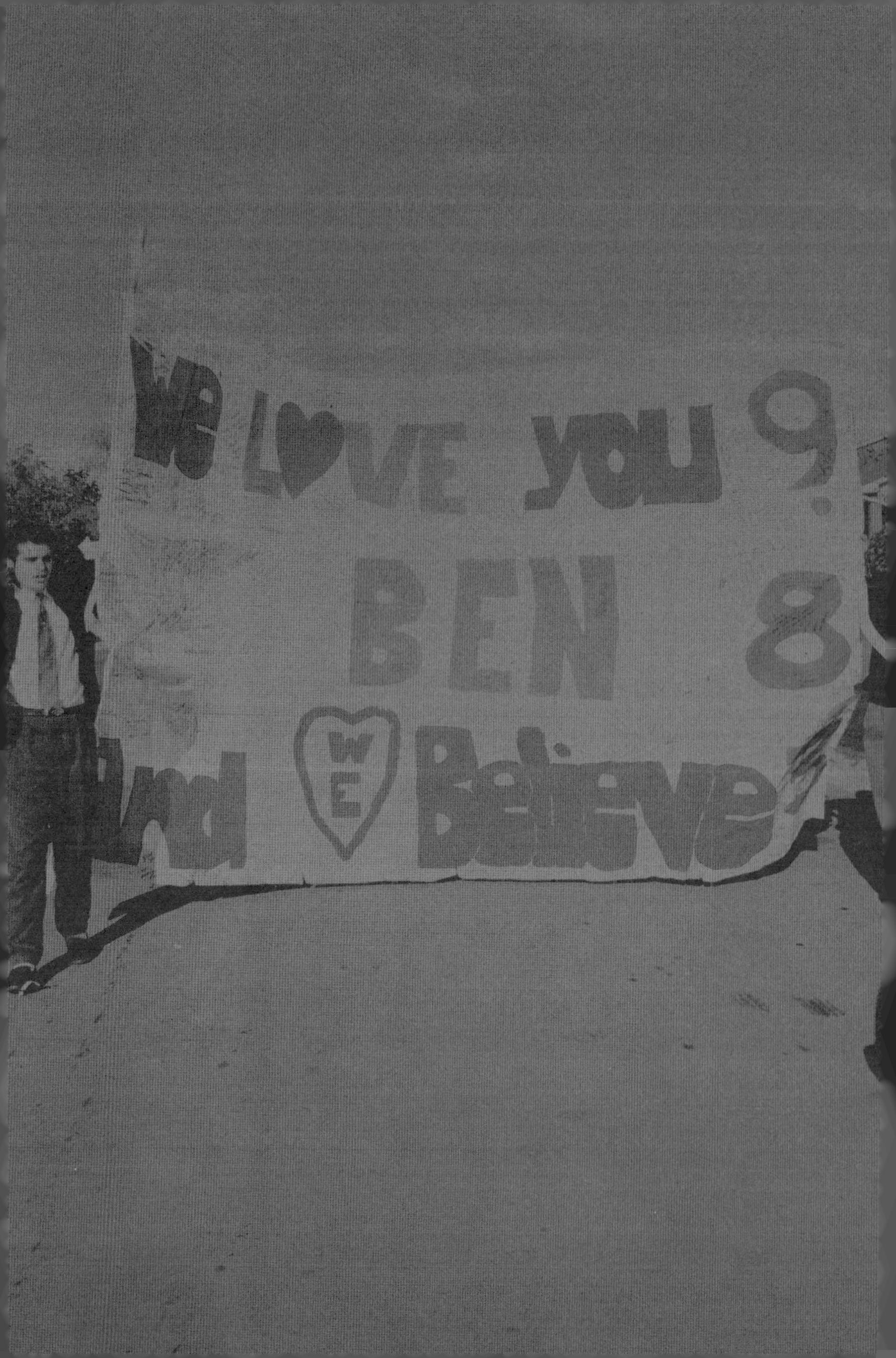
We LOVE YOU 9
BEN 8
And WE Believe

CHAPTER 5

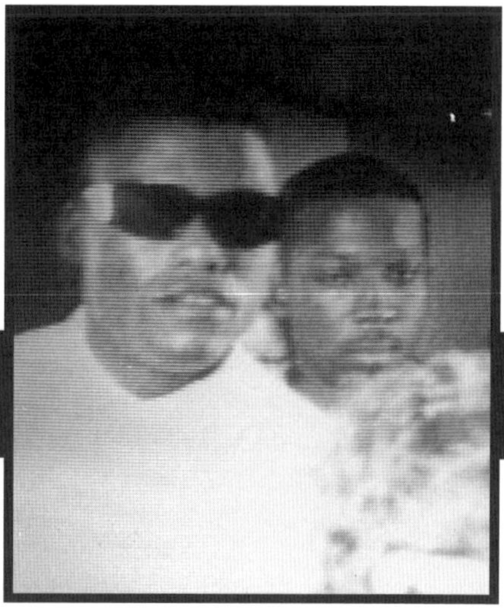

"The Mystery Man" Comes Forward

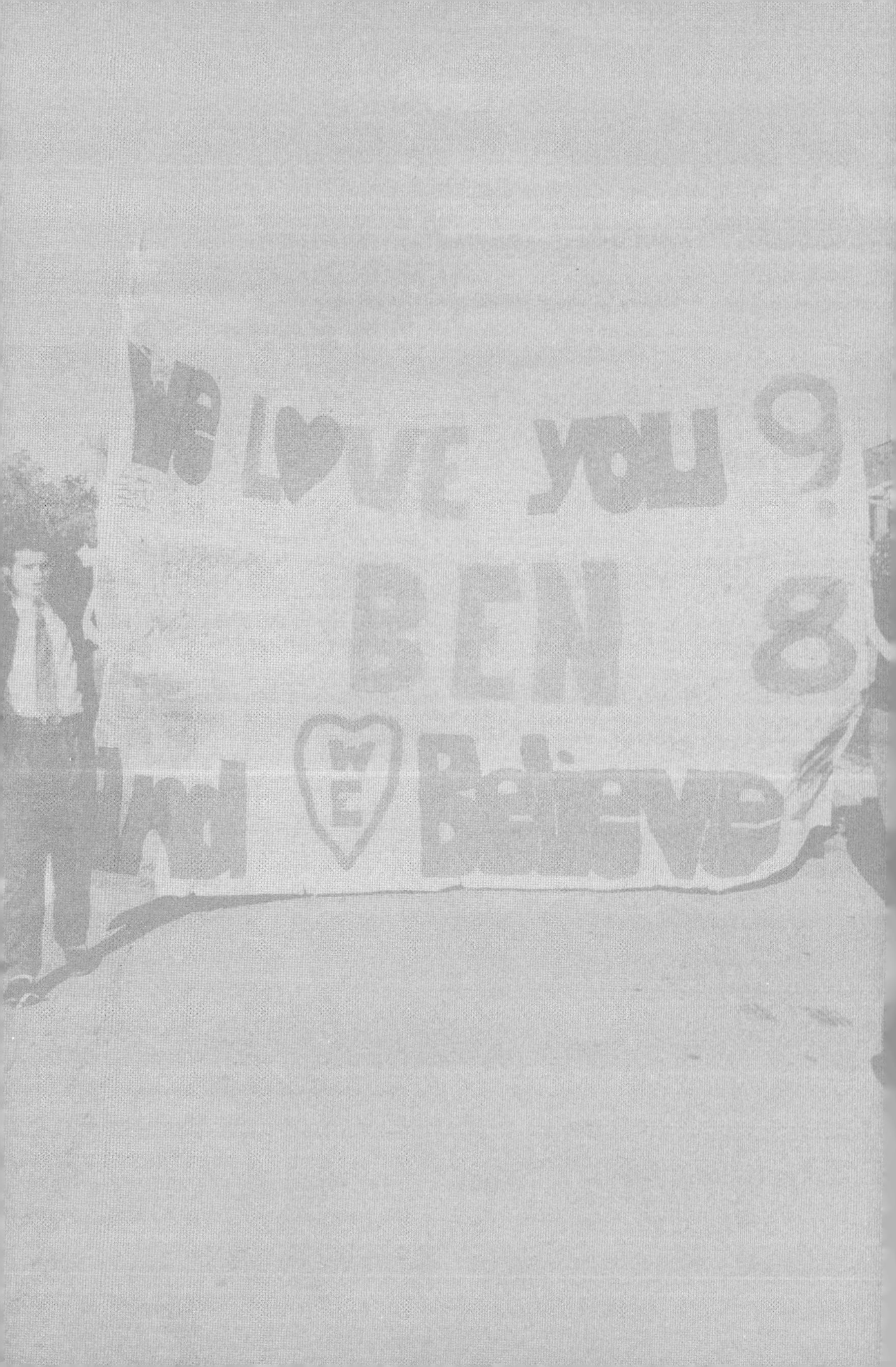
We Love you 9
BEN 8
WE
Believe

CHAPTER 5

"The Mystery Man" Comes Forward

It was not until 2004 that the air began to clear for me. I had suspected all along that I had been cheated in Seoul. In September, my suspicions of being set up were confirmed. A friend and I flew to Los Angeles, California to meet with André Jackson. André had called, requesting this meeting. He wanted to talk about something very important. The last time I met him, our meeting did not go very well.

The last time I saw André was during his stopover in Toronto in 1995. He had called me and said he wanted to talk to me. I was intrigued by his call and agreed to meet him at Lester B. Pearson International Airport. I was very suspicious. I had not seen André since that day in the doping room in Seoul in 1988. So, I called a friend to come with me. We had planned to secretly record the conversation. But when André saw I was not alone, he seemed annoyed. Perhaps he noticed my friend was very anxious. He spoke to us for a few minutes. Then, he made a quick exit, uttering some profanity. His parting comment to me was sharp, bitter and cruel: "I got you, motherfucker," were his exact words as he left Toronto. Why would he say that if he were not somehow involved in the set up? I had not seen nor heard from him after that until September 2004.

Even though our last meeting was not very cordial, I wanted very much to go to Los Angeles and find out what André had to tell me. However, I was faced with a dilemma: My mother was in the hospital, diagnosed with terminal cancer, given only days to live. I was torn. I did not want to leave my mother's bedside, a vigil I had been keeping for weeks. I could not tell her I was leaving. I sought guidance from my mother's pastor. He told me I should go to Los Angeles. He believed she would understand and know it was important. There was nothing I could do for her and he believed she would have wanted me to go.

After my friend and I landed at the airport in LA, I immediately telephoned André. I was very anxious to meet him, find out what he had to say and get back home. He promised to meet my friend and me at our hotel in a couple of hours. At this point, it was still a mystery why he had called this meeting and what he wanted to impart. But I was excited and very curious. He would not have asked me to fly to LA unless it was important. I could not wait for his arrival.

When André arrived at the hotel around 2:00 p.m., he called me from the front desk to get my room number. Eager to see him, I opened my hotel room door and watched him walk down the hall toward me. As he approached, I noticed he was carrying something: a case of beer. As always, he greeted me as if we were old friends, just as he had done after the race in Seoul. We all sat down. He reached for a beer from the case he was carrying and asked if I wanted one. It was déjà vu. I was extremely keen to hear what André had to say but I did not want to appear anxious.

At first, we just exchanged pleasantries, chatting about our "friendship," when we first met and what had been happening since. André had done well for himself. He had acquired an African diamond mine in the Congo. I was very intrigued. The story behind how he had acquired the diamond mine was even more fascinating.

While he was attending university in Southern California, André said he roomed with the son of the Prime Minister of the Congo at that time. Unfamiliar with his newfound freedom and influenced by the LA lifestyle, the Congolese young man started to neglect his studies, staying out late at night and hanging around with the wrong crowd. André stepped in, taking the young man under his wing.

Through this relationship, André was invited to accompany his roommate back to Africa to spend the Christmas holidays with his affluent family. André then reminisced about how he sat for hours talking to his roommate's father, a man who was very eager to know everything about the United States of America. During that conversation, the Prime Minister apparently told André that North American cars, especially the Cadillac, interested him. The Prime Minister expressed a desire to own one. The following Christmas, as a gift to the Prime Minister, André bought and shipped to the Congo a brand new Cadillac. In return for this generous gift, the Congolese government gave André the deed to a small diamond mine.

I was impressed by André's story, but my impatience was beginning to mount. I wanted to know what it was that André had called me all this way to talk about. I was becoming very edgy and feeling guilty about leaving my sick mother in Toronto. I wanted to get back to her as soon as possible. I just could not stop wondering about her and still felt conflicted about being in LA. He had to get to the point and soon. So, I asked André directly why he wanted me to come to Los Angeles.

He told me he wanted to discuss the events surrounding the 1988 Seoul Olympics and my positive test results. From then on, the conversation that followed was, at times, much like a chess game, mentally tiring and frustrating. He spoke in riddles, telling me a piece of the story, and then pausing to ask a question about my own recollection of events. As I spoke, he would add bits and pieces, and then ask another question, as if trying to direct me to where he wanted to take the conversation. It was mentally and emotionally exhausting, but I persisted because I was so eager to know more.

André reflected back to May 31, 1986 in San Jose, when I had problems checking into my hotel before the Bruce Jenner Classic. There had been no reservation made under my name and they had no rooms available. I recalled this incident. I had waited in the lobby of the hotel for almost four hours until the meet promoters arrived to clear up the confusion so I could get into my room.

André said the Lewis camp orchestrated this in an attempt to aggravate me and put me off my game. He said this incident with my hotel room marked the beginning of their attempts to sabotage me. Despite their efforts in San Jose, I was still triumphant. Despite my fatigue, I beat Carl Lewis.

According to André, Lewis was very upset and bothered that their tactic to wear me out had failed. André confirmed that this was, in fact, the turning point when Lewis and his crew would begin to focus more attention on me. Their goal was to find a way to change the outcome of our races in Lewis's favour.

André claimed the same tactics were used in June 1986 at the Goodwill Games in Moscow. Again, I won the race, another defeat for Lewis. My time was 9.95 seconds, the fastest time ever at sea level. It was also a personal best for me. After the race, the media descended on Lewis looking for an explanation for his loss. "What happened, King Carl?" they wanted to know.

Lewis and I were to compete next in Zürich on August 13, 1986. André asked me how much I recalled about a conversation he and I had on the day of that race. We had driven together to the track in the same courtesy car. I remembered that I had talked to him that day. He reminded me how he had befriended me. He had caught my attention by suggesting we go out to a club after the race, saying he already had a couple of girls lined up. He described how warm it had been when we arrived at the track and how he hung around me while I warmed up. He asked me if I remembered him bringing me some water. I did recall this and that I drank from the bottle as I warmed up. I ran the race and placed first, beating Carl Lewis for the third straight time. André revealed this was when the plan to sabotage me in Seoul was formulated.

André went on to describe how he continued to win my trust by befriending me. After the Zürich race, he had called me up to invite me out to the nightclub, as we had discussed earlier that day. I decided to go and celebrate my win. We met in the lobby of the hotel and went to the Ritz Nightclub. On the way, André told me he had three girls lined up for us. I jokingly told him I wanted the best looking one. When we arrived at the club, the champagne was already flowing and André proceeded all night to pour me drink after drink. André said this was a test to see how trusting and observant I was. He also confirmed that the champagne was spiked with stanozolol and that this night was meant to seal our friendship for future chances to stay close to me.

As he continued to share his confession, André became more relaxed, almost jovial. He frankly and boldly told us the whole thing was a setup orchestrated by Carl

Lewis and his entourage. He went so far as to say Carl made reference to the scheme in his book, Inside Track. André noted that Carl's book recounted André's evening with me at the Ritz. He said Carl mocked me by pointing out how André and I had both been interested in the same girl, but André had gotten her phone number and I had not. That is not how I remember the evening. But that's okay. It does not matter. André told me I was very high on the Lewis Camp's radar after Zürich. And he said they were prepared to do whatever it took to take me down.

The next meeting between Carl and me was in Rome. It was August 30, 1987 at the World Championships. To avoid any accommodation problems, as I had experienced in the past, I chose to stay in a hotel rather than the Olympic Village where most of the other athletes were staying. I made sure Larry confirmed my own private reservations ahead of time. On my first day of training at the Olympic Village, I heard that Lewis was already making comments in the media, claiming he thought I was using something to enhance my ability. Lewis went on to declare that, as far as he was concerned, I had come out of nowhere, beating him in the last three races. André confirmed that the plan in Rome was simply to discredit me, to arouse suspicion and to put me under the microscope. Nothing else was done in Rome, according to André, except to plant the seed of doubt in the minds of the media. By putting me and my achievements in doubt and linking me with steroid use, their plan for the 1988 Olympics was well underway.

André was now toying with my memory, asking me to recall the day before the men's 100 metre heats in Seoul. I remember the races well and some events prior to the competition. I remember Charlie and me training in the tent, working out on the warm-up track. I remember there was a massage table and a fridge containing water bottles. I also remember André being at the track, already there when we arrived. I remember him greeting me, as an old friend would. André also remembered these things, describing them to me vividly. He, too, remembered the Canadian delegation tent with its tables, water bottles and other supplies. He admitted he deliberately avoided going into the tent where I was. He did not want to be around Charlie. He felt Charlie would have most likely been suspicious of him.

The plan that day, according to André, was to put something in my water bottle. He brazenly admitted the intent was to set me up for a positive test, to place a steroid in my system that would metabolize and suggest long-term use. He went on to say they wanted to use something strong that would show prominently in my urine test. I listened coolly to these revelations. I had already accepted years ago that I was set up. But to hear it being laid out so calculatingly was chilling.

On a roll now, André admitted administering the steroid to me on that day. He had made his move when I was finished at the warm-up track and away from Charlie. I was in the weight room doing bench presses when André carried out his deed. He said this is how the steroid was planted in my system in advance of the finals, long enough time for the steroid to build up and be detectable in my system. Holding back nothing, André further admitted to purchasing the steroids in Texas, transporting them in his carry-on luggage and being nervous while clearing customs in Seoul.

But the scheme was not yet completed. After the meeting at the warm-up track, I did not see André for the rest of the day. His avoidance of me was deliberate that day. Later that evening when I returned to the hotel, I called my mother. She told me she had dreamed of a snake biting me on the leg. Again, she warned me about eating or drinking anything suspicious. Then she told me to just get some rest and not worry too much about it. I did just that and tried to put it out of my mind. But now, as André was telling me the full detail, everything that happened to me in Seoul began to fall frighteningly into place.

The rest of the time in Seoul, especially before the finals, André said he would seek me out to check on me, almost like a spy. After the semifinals, approximately two hours before the final, I was sleeping in the tent on the warm-up track. André came by the tent when I was alone, I presumed, to talk to me. I did not know he was simply monitoring me, making sure their plans were unfolding successfully, as he described it to me now.

André's outpouring of confessions continued. I say confessions because that is what he called it. He told me it had been bothering him all these years. He spoke of his sense of guilt and needing to get it off his chest. He said he now wanted to help me understand exactly what had happened. He wanted to move on. He must have known that I wanted to move on as well.

What he was telling me was not good news. Neither was it new to me: I had suspected sabotage from day one but no one would listen to me. However, it was a relief to hear his admission of responsibility and get confirmation that what I had known and had been saying all along was true: I had been set up. His words would help me to close out a chapter in my life and help me to understand more completely what had happened to me in Seoul and why.

André did not say how he got into the testing room and I did not ask. But we both knew his presence there was inappropriate. In Carl's book, he speculates that André must have taken one of the American security passes. In any event, André was already in the room when I arrived. He was sitting on the ground next to the fridge, with an American team identification tag hanging from his neck. Meanwhile, this room was neither for the Americans, nor for runners-up. It was reserved for the winner, the gold medalist. I asked him why he was there. At the time, André explained that he was there to congratulate me. Sixteen years later in a hotel room in LA, he was owning up to having been there for other reasons.

While I was in the waiting room, stretched out on the table for my massage, André said he was watching with keen attention. He paid particular interest to who was coming into and going out of the room. From his position seated on the floor in front of the bench, André was able to take full advantage of the situation. He knew I was thirsty and dehydrated and would soon have to provide a urine sample. He also knew I would welcome a drink. He was very happy to oblige. He could also observe that I was in pain as I lay there, face down, wincing with each pressure applied by Waldemar. André admitted this was when he had the opportunity to reach inside a Mizuno pouch he wore around his waist to retrieve the stanozolol. According to him, the pouch was full of stanozolol pills, the same ones he had transported to Seoul in his carry on from Texas. According to André, he deposited one capsule into each beer that I drank. I consumed eight beers. This would explain why they found stanozolol in my urine test. The pills must have dissolved fairly quickly. I did not recall any taste. I did remember feeling buzzed. André remembered, too.

It was about this time that the photographs later published in Carl's book were taken. The first one is of André sitting on the floor in front of me, as I lay on the bench, beer cans on the floor. The caption under this photo reads, "My friend André Jackson with Ben Johnson in the drug-testing area at the 1988 Seoul Games. At the time, André had no idea he would be labeled, 'The Mystery Man.'" The second photograph was taken of André, Diane Clement, who was holding my gold medal, and me. After these pictures were taken, André simply got up and left the room without saying a word. His deed was done.

As I listened intently to this man, I kept getting flashbacks: the USA identification card around his neck, his association with Carl Lewis, the beers, the Mizuno pouch. What did all this mean? I understood that I had played into a trap, but by whom and for what? According to André, he did not really believe that Carl was completely apprised of the plan in Seoul. But there were others in Lewis's camp who definitely knew what was going on. André even hinted that there were many clues about the scheme included in Carl's book. He encouraged me to read the book because it held so many important links: Just read between the lines and you will be able to connect the dots from what I have told you.

To emphasize his point, André again referred back to the photographs taken in the doping room in Seoul. Mizuno was to be Carl's major sponsor after the Seoul Olympics. André emphasized that a win for Carl would have sky-rocketed the sales of Mizuno shoes. André said he himself was wearing Mizuno shoes at the time. Was he implicating Mizuno? He would not come right out and say it. But he gave another hint: He told us to look at the next picture in Carl's book. Carl and his teammates posed for an endorsement photograph to promote Mizuno. Each one of them is holding a Mizuno shoe, prominently marked with the company logo.

I have, of course, spoken with Bryan, my spiritual advisor, about this meeting with André Jackson and his confession. Through his gift, Bryan discerned that Carl was not involved, directly or indirectly, in planning my sabotage. I know this is true. And based on this Truth, I cannot blame Carl Lewis. However, I am hoping that Carl will shed some light on what knowledge he might have in connection to my sabotage. On some level, both Carl and I became casualties of the official rulings that followed the final race in Seoul: Carl won the gold medal with many people doubting he won it fairly and I lost the gold medal with many people feeling I was treated unfairly.

André talked about the elusive "Mystery Man" mentioned by the media after the Seoul fiasco. He and I both knew there was no mystery. But none of the officials even bothered to investigate the sabotage theory, nor did the Dubin Inquiry, despite all of the journalists' questions about a "Mystery Man."

The day after the gold medal 100 metre race, André hopped on a plane and disappeared. He would follow the aftermath of my ordeal from a safe distance. As soon as he heard about the Dubin Inquiry, he went even further into hiding, fearing he may be called as a witness. He left the United States for Africa where he stayed for almost a year. He returned a few months after the Dubin Inquiry had concluded when the dust had settled. He simply carried on with his life.

Why was André coming forward with this information now? He just wanted to help me and clear his mind, he said. I was stunned and angry to hear him recount the plot to smear my name and orchestrate my downfall, although at the same time, I was to some extent relieved and heartened to finally know the truth. My mother's discernment was starting to come to pass. I was simultaneously gratified and dumbfounded. It was almost unbelievable.

Was André prepared to go public, disclose this information to the media and clear my name? He said he would not go directly to the media with me, but would confirm the facts if called upon. He wanted to clear the air for me and clear his conscience, then move on with his life. Through discernment, Bryan confirmed that André's soul is fearful of disclosing certain information that would help to exonerate me. Bryan also told me that God would show favouritism to André if he does come forward publicly and speak the truth.

Why did André do this to me? A matter of putting bread and butter on the table, he told my friend and me. He said he did it for the American team and for great personal financial benefit. Was it Mizuno who had paid him? He would neither confirm nor deny this. Instead, he stated, in a matter of fact way: the pouch he was wearing that day, which he had filled with stanozolol, was given to him directly by a Mizuno senior executive and Mizuno was Carl's sponsor.

André's story and assertions need further exploration in order to assist in clearing my name. I call upon everyone who was connected to my disqualification, including Mr. André Jackson, to step forward and either support or dispel this story. I have nothing to hide.

Did André realize what he had done had almost ruined my life? Yes, he did. Why didn't he confess sooner, like in 1995 when we met at the Toronto airport? When the Dubin Inquiry was over, André said he felt confident he would never be found out: He was just passing through and wanted to gloat. In addition, he answered that he could not confess. He was still involved with Lewis's people on some business deals. In playing a key role in my sabotage, the result was not only a gold medal for Lewis, but a financial gain for many around him as well.

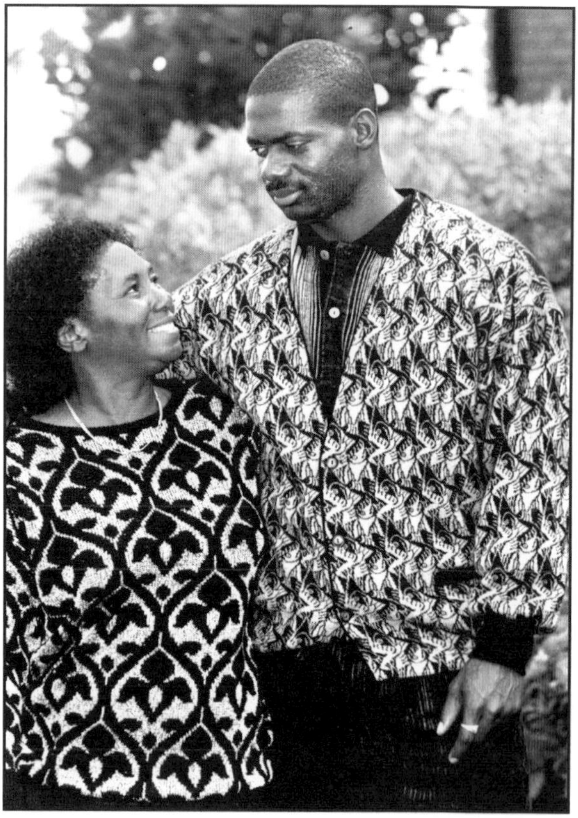

After my visit with André in California, I was drained. I needed to process the information I received. I secluded myself in my LA hotel room. My thoughts were in a tailspin... the assaults from the media, the criticisms by the Canadian government, the unforgiving spirit of sports administrators... Why? What did I do to deserve this misfortune? How could someone do this to me for money? Why would someone go to this extent to sabotage me, simply for their own gain? I could not understand. My career had been derailed, my family disgraced. I felt like the wind was knocked right out of me. The weight of the information André gave me was crushing. I was reminded, all over again, of the humiliation I felt in Seoul and the devastation I experienced during the Dubin Inquiry.

As I was packing for my return flight home, the news came. The phone rang. It was my sister in Toronto. My mother had just passed away. On hearing this, I fell down on the couch and sobbed uncontrollably. I could not gather my thoughts. I wanted so much to share with her what André had told me. But now I would not get that opportunity. The second part of my mother's discernment had also come to pass: She would not be here to see me clear my name.

My mother was the most important person in the world to me and now she was gone. I could not imagine going home and not having her greet me at the door. She was a constant and serene haven during all my nightmares. She often spoke to me about God's Will. Whenever something bad happened, it was God's Will, she would say. We should not challenge it. She told me Seoul was a small piece of God's puzzle for my life. She told me to maintain my faith in God. I have always had a deep respect and admiration for my mother. Now that she was gone, I just sat and accepted that all of this was the Will of God.

My mother had made her wishes clear. She wanted to be buried in Canada close to her children. The procession from the church we attended together regularly to the cemetery was the hardest day of my life. Not Seoul. Not the Dubin Inquiry. Not André's confession. Nothing compared to this loss. I flashed back to the day she left Jamaica for Canada, leaving me behind. Now, I was left behind again. Traditionally, Jamaican men are very close to and protective of their mothers. There is a saying in Jamaica: When you lose your mother, the person who brought you into this world, it is only then that you become a man, no longer a son.

The funeral was well attended. I was proud of her. I live to make her proud of me. It was going to be very rough. I had no choice but to carry on.

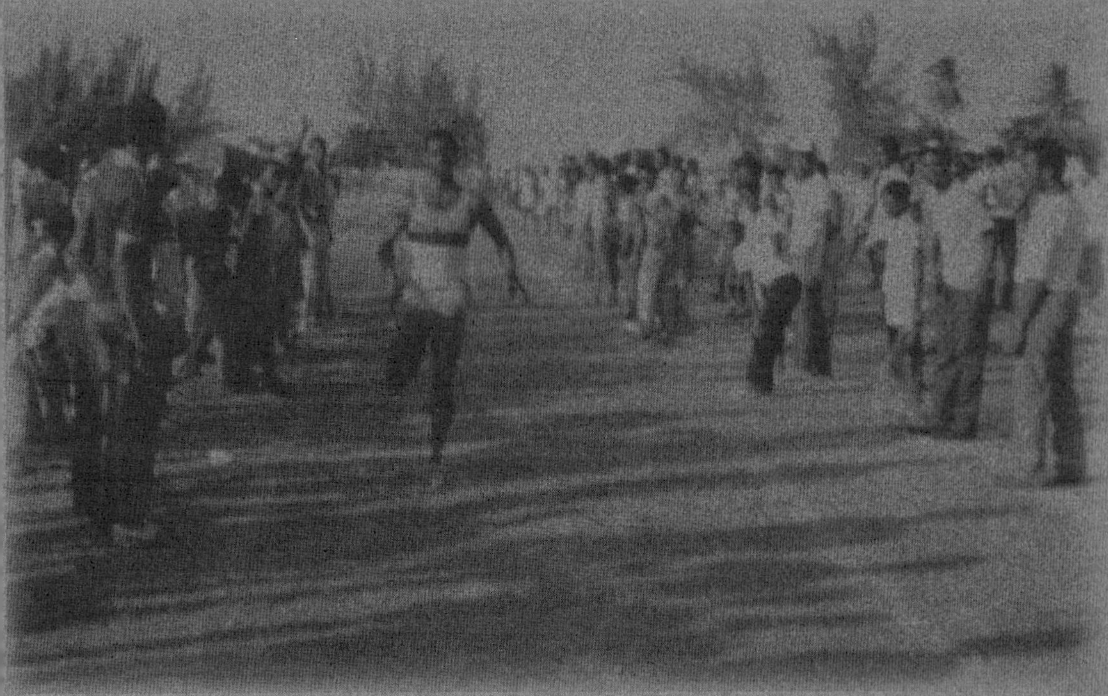

CHAPTER 6

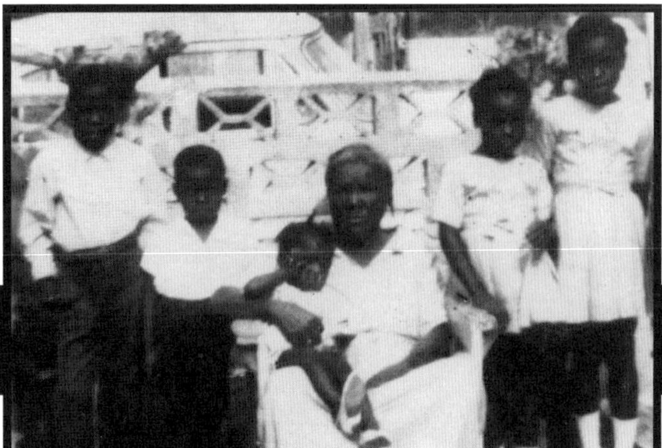

Born in Jamaica with the Desire to Win

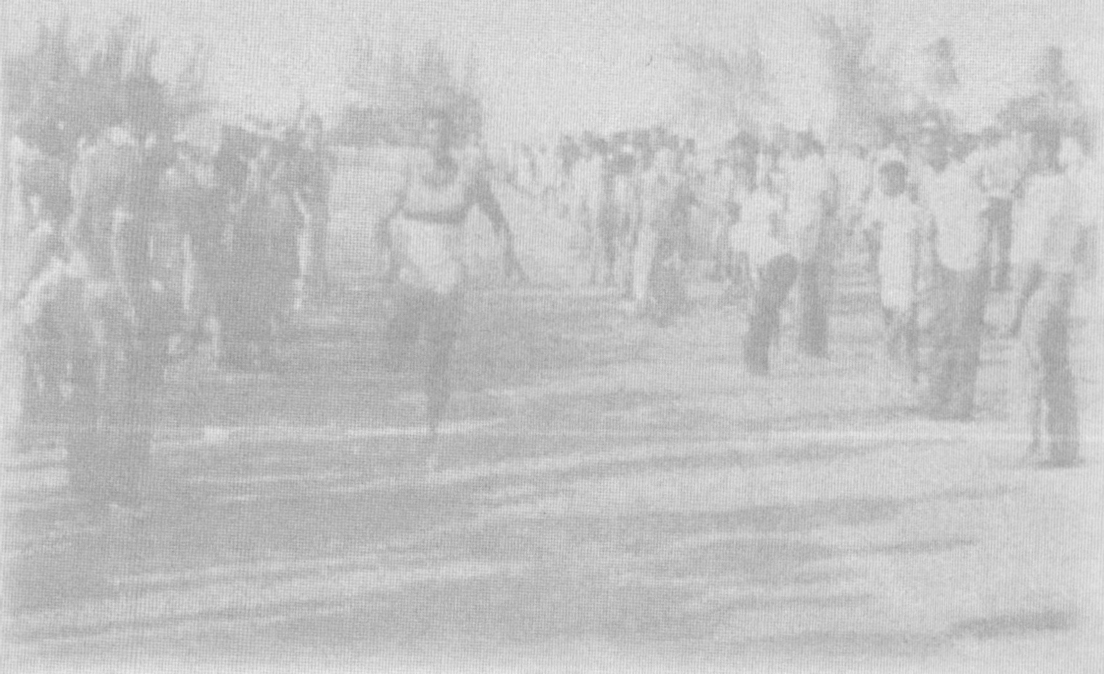

CHAPTER 6

Born in Jamaica with the Desire to Win

My mother, Gloria, was a beautiful woman of Jamaican/Cuban descent while my father, Ben Sr., was Jamaican. My parents met when my mother was 16 and my father was 26. My grandfather, Aubrey Case, opposed the union due to the ten-year age difference. However, my father was very determined, a trait I like to think we share. He frequently appeared at the Case house on the pretense of speaking with my mother's older brothers. Over time, my Grandfather Case got to know Benjamin and found he was a hard worker. He soon realized the young couple was in love and consented to their marriage. They married in September 1952, making their home in Falmouth, a few miles east of Montego Bay.

In addition to sea and sun, and its history of sugar and rum, slavery and ships, Falmouth is known for its fish, jerk pork and easy life, not unlike other places in Jamaica. But nowhere else had the Martha Brae, the emerald coloured river, meandering its way slowly past the town, providing scenic beauty and rafting experiences and attracting people from all over the world, near and far, from all walks of life. At the point where the river empties out into the ocean, the Martha Brae passes through a mangrove, creating a magical effect that makes the water glisten with a flickering light.

According to legend, Martha Brae was an old witch of Arawak descent, the original people of Jamaica. As the story goes, she lived by the river and was captured by the Spaniards who hoped to use her as a guide to find Arawak gold. Pretending to be helpful, she led them to one of the caves lining the river and suddenly disappeared. Frightened, the Spaniards ran but the river swallowed them up. It is said Martha Brae then used her powers to change the course of the river to hide the gold from discovery.

We grew up listening to this story and I always wondered if it was true. So, I asked Bryan to ask God about Martha Brae.

Ben, you ask Me about a woman, a witch, a human being of great powers who is known as Martha Brae. Did such a person exist? Yes, this person did exist. And yes, she did have certain abilities to look into the future and to know things about others. But let Me tell you: You are not to admire her; the people of Jamaica are not to worship such a person. For this one, her powers were used to have power over others, to cause people to do things against their will. For she only wished to look after herself, first, last and always... Oh yes, she claimed to know Me. She claimed to know My Son, Jesus. She claimed to know the Heavens. She claimed many things. But she was not of Truth. She was not of Me. For I say to My Children: Be wary of those who have spiritual gifts, who claim to be of Me, but are not able to confirm Truth on a yea, yea; nay, nay basis.

Bryan paused. I looked at him and he closed his eyes again. God continued:

Ben, for the people of Jamaica are trapped by those who do witchcraft, by those who do voodoo and, yes, by those who claim to speak in tongues. For very few who speak in tongues are of Me. For you will know: The ones who speak in tongues who are of Me are also able to confirm Truth on a yes, yes or no, no basis. For those whom I work through always love and always forgive unconditionally.

Ben, for many of My Children have been hurt badly around the world by the so-called fortune tellers. Many of these who claim to be of Me have powers to be able to curse another, to be able to bring disease into another. For I say to all My Children: Be careful with all the false beliefs that can weigh you down, that can cause you to give your power away to another. My Children have been given free will, but it has been compromised by their false beliefs. My Children need to purify their souls and let go of these false beliefs that limit, that restrict them, at times, from having free will. For all My Children: be careful what you believe in. Trust only in Me.

After getting married, my parents immediately began family life together. My parents' first child was Dezrine, my father's daughter from a previous relationship. My mother raised Dezrine as one of her own. Clare came next, followed by Edward, then Jean, and then another son named Norman. Sadly, Norman contracted a childhood illness and died. This was a very traumatic event for the young family.

I was born on December 30, 1961. My parents named me Benjamin Sinclair Johnson, Jr. after my father. They were ecstatic that I was healthy. But three weeks after I was born, the village of Falmouth was overcome with malaria. Many of the newborn infants were infected, including me. Determined not to lose another child, my mother held me in her arms constantly for six months, nursing me back to health and praying for my survival. She breast fed me and gave me lemonade to fight dehydration. She prayed, begged, and bargained with God to save me.

I know that God heard my mother's prayers because I am here today. I survived. My mother told me this was a miracle; this was a sign I was destined for something special. Bryan has since confirmed this. He discerned that my personal records in God's Archives show that it was by Divine intervention that I survived. Many of the other children affected did not make it, but I did. I am thankful.

About a year and a half later, my mother gave birth to my younger sister, Marcia. She is called Junie by her friends and family, as it is quite traditional in Jamaica to be given a pet name. Junie became her name because she was born in June. Junie was my first playmate. When she became old enough, I would fight with her and then take off. She would retaliate by throwing a stone at me with the accuracy of an American League pitcher.

Junie threw stones at me out of frustration. At times, I did not pick up after myself and she would end up cleaning up instead. Another reason why she threw stones at me was because she believed, at times, I had made fun of her. I do agree I should have cleaned up, but making fun of other people is not part of who I am. From my point of view, it seemed like she sometimes misconstrued what I was actually saying.

I asked Bryan to discern this. He confirmed it is true. He said that I learned two important lessons about women through this experience. The first lesson: do not underestimate how a woman will respond. And the second: be very careful with how you treat a woman. Showing unconditional love goes a long way.

My father was very industrious and worked hard to support his young family. He worked as a technician for the Jamaica Public Service (JPS), a utility company supplying electricity and telephone service to the Island. On weekends, he operated a limousine service for the tourist industry, driving a big white Chevrolet Bel Air. He also had a bee nursery in our backyard and sold honey. During his 40 years of employment, only on very rare occasions did he take sick leave or miss a day of work for any reason at all. Such was his desire and ability to overcome any obstacle.

My mother stayed at home to raise the family and tend to her large garden of both vegetables and flowers. My mother loved plants of all kinds and the variety that could be grown on the Island was magnificent. My mother was a very proud, strong, self-confident, compassionate and spiritually gifted woman. She had a very caring and gentle heart. She also had a great sense of humour. To say my mother was spiritual means she encouraged all our family members to take full accountability and responsibility for our own actions, or lack of actions, and she encouraged us, when things went wrong, not to blame others and not to blame God. She also encouraged me and others to love and forgive unconditionally, not to accept "Eye for an eye," not to accept or act out revenge on another.

Much has been said about how hard it was to live on the Island. But that is not what I remember as a child growing up. My family was middle class by Jamaican standards. My parents believed in hard work, that nothing comes easy. They also valued sharing and gave generously to others. Many times, I remember my father coming home with boxes of provisions that my mother would then share with needy children from the streets.

I remember mostly laughter and lively, lighthearted chatter, the warm sun beating down on my skin, the sound of waves washing up on rocky and sandy shores, the smell of fish and salt, and the feel of the ocean breeze hitting my face as my friends and I splashed and swam in the open sea. These are my fondest childhood memories. I remember my mother's happiness with her friends, the singing and praying in church, my father's JPS van, his bees and hard work.

As a child, I was somewhat intimidated by my father, a very tall and strong man. He was definitely the disciplinarian in our family. When he raised his voice we all stopped in our tracks. Even so, I enjoyed spending time with him. Many people in Falmouth respected my father as a community leader. He would often conduct town meetings with the men of the village to discuss local politics and issues. Many times, I would sit for hours listening to my father talk to other men in the community about current events. I also recall spending many hours on weekends with my father, as he would drive around to deliver his honey and visit friends. During our long car rides, my father would talk to me about life lessons, instilling his wisdom in me.

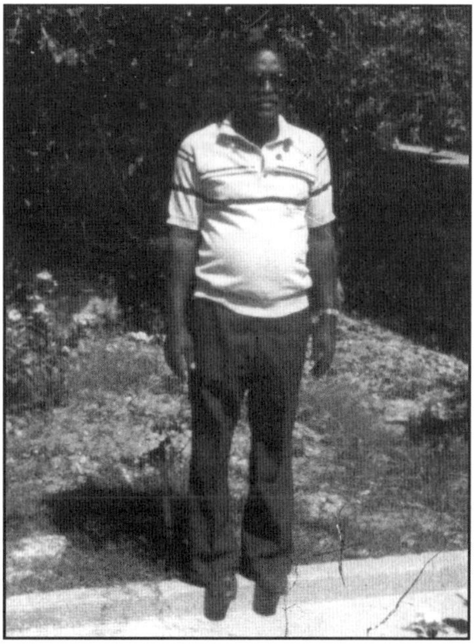

Because of my illness as a child, both of my parents were highly protective of me. My siblings would probably concur that my mother favoured me and spoiled me a bit. But she would say she tried to treat all her children equally. My father balanced that with high expectations. He was a strict and stern disciplinarian across the board with all the children.

I asked Bryan about raising children and the biblical idea of "sparing the rod and spoiling the child." Is it God's Will for parents to discipline children harshly?"

Ben, you ask the question about sparing the rod. The question remains in the hearts, in the minds of many. Is it My Will for a parent to scold, to beat their children? This belief is in place, based on the many false beliefs that man has brought forward from one incarnation to the next. It is not My Will for any child to be disciplined in such a way that he or she will never forget that moment, that day of being harmed.

It is true: For a child to be beaten is an act of betrayal, on some level, by the one who is doing the beating. They do not understand how to give love. They are not connected to their heart, and unable to know Truth. If they were truly connected to their heart, they would be able to call upon Me for the answer. For they have false beliefs that they must beat their children due to fear of being weak in front of their children, in front of others.

All of My Children: Forgive the children, your children who do wrong. Understand your children. Do not be quick to react. Look into the child's eyes and you will see the mirror. For that which disturbs you in the child must be healed within you. Once you have healed your soul, you will be able to understand how to heal your children. And once you stop judging your children, judging others, you know you are healed. And the harsh discipline only becomes a past memory, soon to be forgotten.

Ben, I ask that you forgive your father for any harm he may have caused you. For the soul of your father and your soul have a great past. And throughout your life, this life, it is your journey to heal your soul. And as your father's soul is healed by you going through the different levels of forgiveness, both of you will become closer each time, removing all that holds both of you from bonding even closer.

I have forgiven my father.

I remember Christmas being particularly exciting, a beautiful time of year for our family, especially for children. But it wasn't about Santa Claus or presents under the tree. It was about time spent together and the feasts of turkey, pig and goat which my father was skilled at preparing. It was about the smell of mother's baking, the sounds of music, and the Jonkonnu masquerade dances in the street. As a boy, I was dreadfully afraid of the Jonkonnu dancers. Whenever I would misbehave, my sisters would threaten to throw me out on the streets to the dancers if I did not listen. No wonder I could run so fast! The girls would have to catch me first.

The Jonkonnu dancers, scary and attractive at the same time, were a special favourite. As I got older and realized the dancers would not harm me, my friends and I would follow them as they paraded through the streets. Masked and dressed in colourful costumes, these men would dance and jig through the streets to the tune of beating drums and a whistling fife or flute. They collected money as they went along. I did not know it then, but the masquerades were carry-overs from African folk culture that survived as a reminder of our heritage. The Horse Head, the Policeman, the Belly Woman and others would frighten us as they came near. We would run away as they sprang at us. But we would give them money just the same. It was great fun.

I spoke to Bryan about Christmas. Through his gift, he reminded me there were three things I did not like about Christmas. The first one: people were forced to give presents, gifts to others, out of a holiday obligation and not always from a position of sincerity. The second issue I had with Christmas: people were forced to come together out of obligation with great reluctance. The third: Christmas often brings jealousy among individuals who are supposed to love each other.

Then Bryan told me how I really view Christmas, on a soul level: a day to be grateful that there is truly a God, if only the world would open up their hearts and receive God. I agree. This is true. This is always how I have felt at the deepest level. I was curious to know more.

So, I asked Bryan to go directly to God and ask Him for more explanation about Christmas. I wondered... what does God have to say about Christmas? The Lord answered:

Ben, you ask the question about Christmas. For each person has their own interpretation of how to celebrate Christmas. Christmas is a time of gathering to rejoice in the spirit of life. It is a time for all to come together and celebrate the breath of life. For not all My Children have this ability, to truly rejoice and receive. Christmas should be a time of spiritual celebration, not so much of material celebration. Many hold such expectations as to what they "want" for Christmas. Instead, they should be thinking only about what they need. In order for the world to become closer to Me, the world must change its course and start living a life based on need and not based on wants.

I gave the world Jesus, the Christ, the true Messiah. He lived by example, to show the world how one can survive on very little, how one can survive by trusting in Me. For the world must realize: The true Gift of Christmas is to be able to say on Christmas Day, each and every day, "I have forgiven all. I have forgiven self. I love and give unconditionally." For this is the True Gift of Christmas. For when one has achieved this level, one can truly say they accept Christ, not before.

At that point, Bryan stopped speaking. I was pondering what God had just said... the true gift of Christmas. Was He saying there is a deeper meaning to accepting Christ?

Ben, many do not understand what it means to accept Christ. There are so many religions, so many teachers. I will take this time, this moment to clarify to My Children what it means to accept Christ. It means to be able to love God with all thy heart, soul, mind and strength. It means to love thy neighbour as thyself. And regardless of who you are, if you can truly do this effortlessly and unconditionally... regardless of your race, your religious beliefs... by default, you will accept Christ. To accept Christ is to walk the talk. It is not about lip service.

Thank You, Father, for answering my long-standing questions and life-long uncertainty about Christmas. And thank You for addressing what it really means to accept Christ.

The streets of Falmouth were my playground. In my neighbourhood, everyone knew each other. They knew where you came from and who your parents were. As I look back now, I realize life was probably difficult in Falmouth. But conversation came easy, laughter was always present, and fun was never hard to come by. As for me, I had few worries, running through the open fields and bushes and splashing in the ocean.

My older brother Edward had a stutter. When I was younger, I used to mock him. At the age of 11, I also developed a stutter which put an end to my mocking! Despite this, I looked up to him. He was a role model for me. He also loved to run. But being older, he was already involved in a local track club. Eventually, Edward earned a track scholarship to a university in Texas.

I proved at a very young age to be extremely determined and competitive. I would often go out of the house to swim, run or go to the movies. One of my favourite activities was to challenge other young boys in the neighborhood to a race. I loved to feel my heart beat and legs strain as I passed the other boys. I won most races. When I was six, I beat one of my friends. After that race, we were no longer friends. This has been a challenge throughout my life: I have often lost friends due to jealousy after winning against them. But back in those days, I was motivated to race because I simply liked the feeling of working hard to win.

At times, other kids would enter a bet with me to race and I remember using my winnings to go to the movies. I would sit and watch movie after movie about far away places and things I had never seen before in Jamaica. Though my parents would often scold me when I eventually came home after being gone all day, it was never enough to deter me.

I loved swimming. In Jamaica, with the beautiful Caribbean Sea and sand, the temptation to spend hours in the water was irresistible to me. Not only would I get in trouble for being gone from the house for so long, I would be in even bigger trouble if my mother found out I was swimming in the sea. Years earlier, three of my uncles were swimming when one became caught in a strong undertow. The other two brothers tried to save him, but ended up losing their lives as well. This heartbreaking event deprived my mother of three of her siblings. Because of this, she was intolerant of my disobedience with regard to swimming. She grounded me many times to no avail.

Often, I would swim with my friends for hours in the Caribbean Sea. I would then spend another hour or so trying to wash the salt from my skin and flush the red from my eyes in an effort to hide from my parents that I had been swimming. Despite the scolding and threat of being grounded, I would still sneak out to join my friends to go to the sea. I could not help myself.

My mother impressed upon me that faith was an integral part of life. She would sit with me at night before bed to say my prayers and read stories from the Bible. From my earliest days, I recall my mother telling me I was a very special little boy and God had saved me for a reason. I grew up believing this to be true, though I had no idea what it meant at the time.

When I was 12, my friend and I were going to the bread shop. My friend was very sick. He could not breathe very well. We were walking on the sidewalk when we saw an old man walking towards us with a bunched up hood on his head and a bag over his shoulders. It seemed like he was lost, looking for something. I remember him stopping us. We gave way to him on the sidewalk as we stepped down into the drainage gutter along the side of the road. He asked for directions but then immediately looked at my friend, asking if he was sick. The old man grabbed my friend's hand and looked at his palm.

At this point, we were getting very nervous. My friend, especially, was becoming really afraid. I could tell from his eyes. It felt as if the old man was getting ready to grab him and take him away. Instead, the old man said to him, "You are very sick. You don't have too much time to live." That made my friend even more afraid. He started crying and then suddenly ran away.

I was too stunned to move. The old man grabbed my left hand and held it out. A chill suddenly came over me. He had told my friend he was going to die. I turned my head. I did not want to hear what he had to tell me. But then, he started speaking, telling me what I would face in the future. He told me I would be traveling around the world. I would be famous. My name would become familiar to many people. But I did not want to hear anymore. As soon as he let go of my hand, I just took off and ran. I looked behind me as I was running. I was very scared.

My friend died a few weeks later, just as the old man said he would. Of course, I told this story of the old man to Bryan. From time to time, I have thought about the old man's prediction and how it came true. I asked Bryan if God would provide me with more information about this man.

Ben, you ask me about the old man who gave you a message, a prediction, based on a vision that he had experienced. For it is not the Will of God for My Children to know the future, for My Children to go to fortune tellers. It is the Will of God for My Children to live in the now, to live in the present, just as I do.

My mother often warned me about fortune tellers but I never asked why. Now that God was telling me this Truth, I was very curious to know why we should not go to fortune tellers. So I asked Bryan to discern the answer. The Lord answered:

My son, you ask a very good question, for My Children have been harmed by fortune tellers. Those who claim to be of Me and predict the future, and foretell the future... for their main purpose is to take you off the path that I have already planned for My Children.

Fortune tellers are very angry at Me. They do not understand Me. They never knew Me. They started out in the beginning with false beliefs, believing that I was a punishing God and believing that they must get even when they are harmed. Fortune tellers have separated themselves from Me, from Truth. For they will provide information for their own benefit, false information that will bring more chaos, more disharmony to one's life, to a family, thus creating a false need by those the fortune tellers harm. Instead of My Children coming to Me when they are in turmoil, they return to the fortune teller until such time the fortune teller has fulfilled its revenge on others.

For My Children have a difficult time walking a path of true spirituality, as many are trapped between being held hostage by fortune tellers and being held hostage through those religions that hold on to false beliefs.

I am glad I asked the question. Thank You, Father.

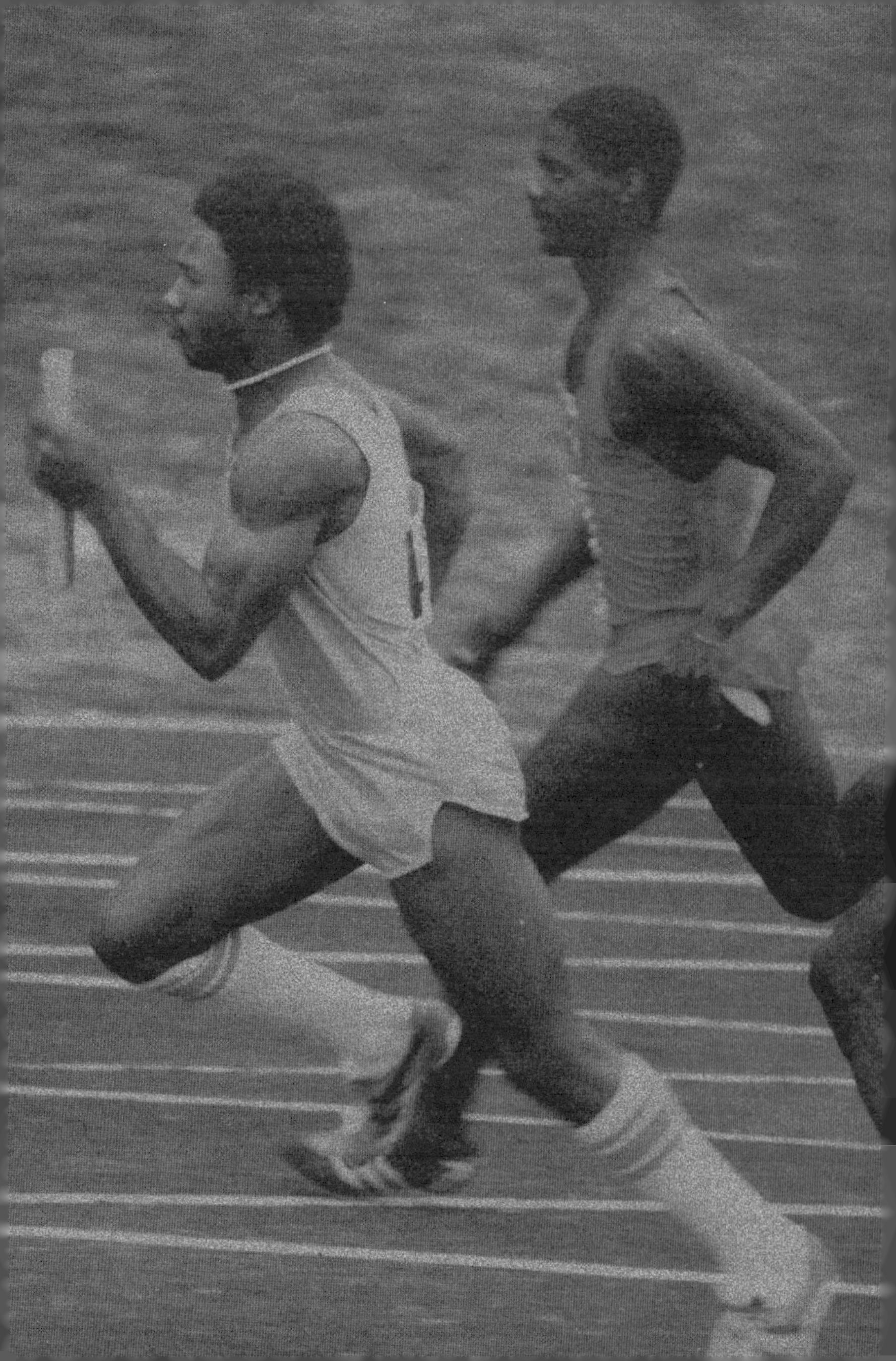

CHAPTER 7

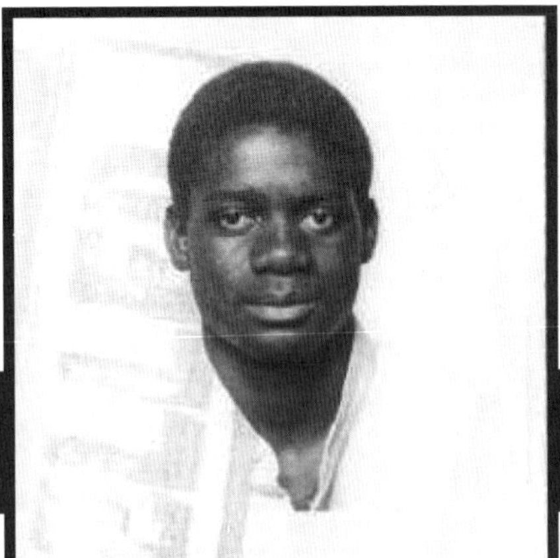

Our New Frontier

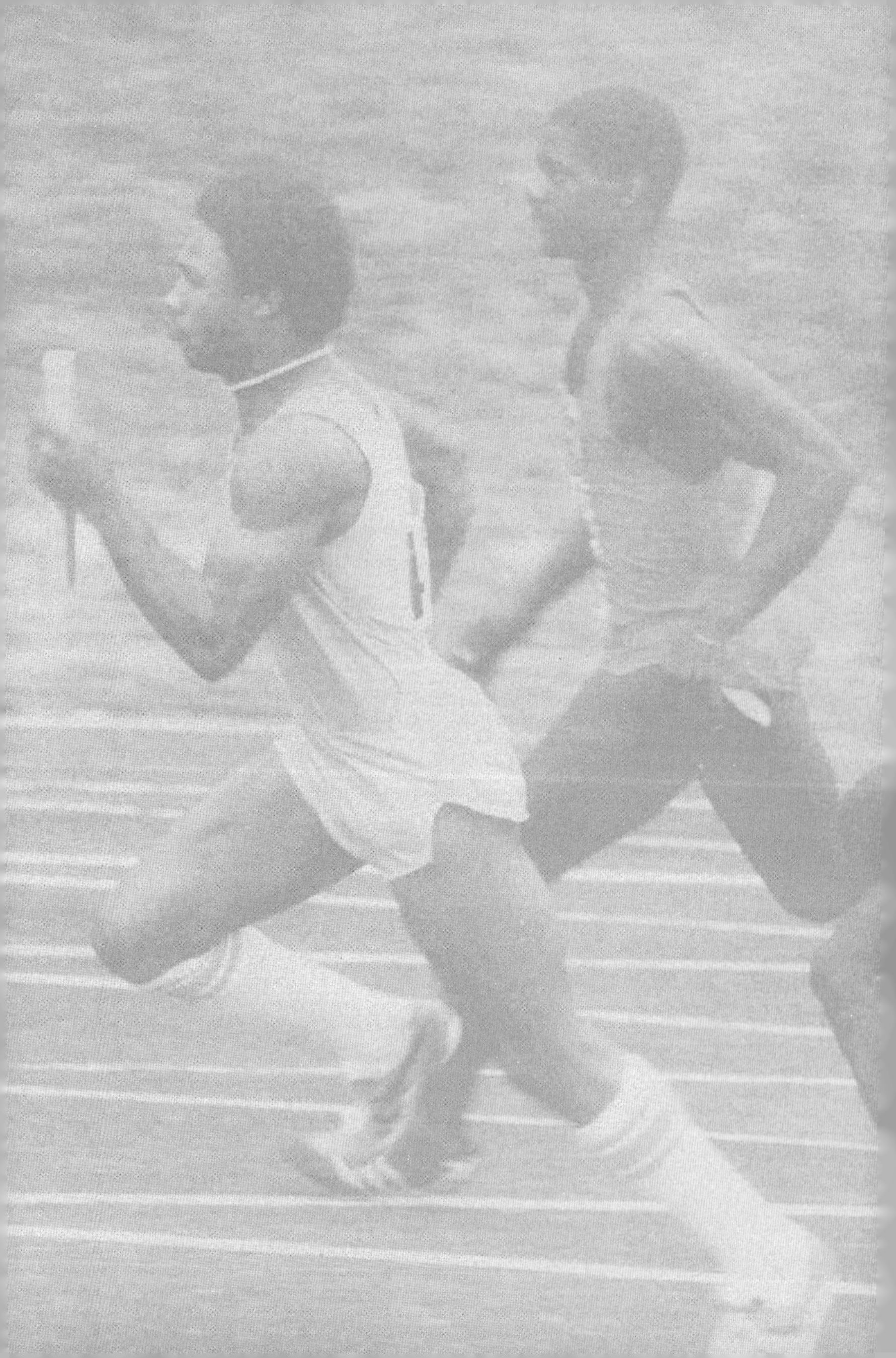

CHAPTER 7

Our New Frontier

In 1972, my mother went to Canada on holiday to visit a girlfriend, Gertrude, who had emigrated from Jamaica. My mother stayed with Gertrude for a couple of weeks and became very impressed with Canada. When she returned to Jamaica, she realized her children could have a much better future in Canada. She discussed the idea with my father and they decided to start taking the steps to move the family to Canada. My father was not entirely in agreement with this but consented to give it a try. He reasoned it would make sense for him to stay in Jamaica and continue to earn a living, supporting the family while she got established. My mother moved to Toronto and stayed with Gertrude temporarily. She soon found employment with a family whose children were hearing-impaired. She worked for them for approximately six months.

I asked Bryan, "Why did God have me end up in Canada, instead of staying in Jamaica?" The Lord answered:

Ben, you ask the question, why did I send you to Canada? For the answer is quite deep, and goes against the many beliefs of My Children who, through one incarnation to the next, hold false beliefs that will not allow them to accept Divine Truth. I sent you to Canada because Canada is a country of old souls. This is a country of many who have had other incarnations of extreme suffering. For through these experiences, on a soul level, they have developed an understanding of why it is important to forgive those who harm you. They have developed an understanding of why it is better to be a peacemaker. You are an old soul. I have sent you to this country to be that peacemaker.

My mother used to say I was here for a reason and God was going to use me to do something great.

The Canadian government, during the Trudeau years, was promoting immigration to Canada. New immigrants who could find full-time employment were allowed to apply for citizenship. My mother took advantage of this program and found a full-time position with Hilton Hotels. She continued to work with the hearing-impaired children as much as possible between her shifts because she had become attached to them. But eventually, she was promoted at the Hilton and could no longer accommodate both. This was her very first job outside of the home. She earned a decent salary, saved her money and received many awards for being an outstanding employee. After about a year, she was able to get her own apartment. But it would be a couple of years before we were reunited.

My mother talked about long-term employment and a better future but I could not see the point of it. The truth is I missed her very much while she was gone. In her absence, our father took care of us, the best way he knew. He did the best he could. But it was not like mother's love. I cried myself to sleep at night and my sisters would fuss over me. But that did not help. My mother was so far away. Through her letters and phone calls, I knew she lived in a place called Toronto. I learned there was something in Toronto called winter with something else called snow. I would go to the local library to read about Canada, just to learn about where she was. From the pictures, I could see there were a lot of white people in Canada. My curiosity and excitement about the place grew. But I still missed my mother. I would not be satisfied until I could be with her again.

My mother only returned to Jamaica to visit a few times during those years. She would tell us stories about Canada and try to convince my father that we would all be very happy there. The immigration and citizenship process in Canada took a lot longer than my mother had originally anticipated. Finally, in April 1976, Edward, Jean, Marcia and I moved to Canada. I was 14 years old. My father, Dezrine and Clare stayed in Jamaica.

My mother came to meet us at the airport with hugs for all of us and tears in her eyes. My uncle on my father's side, Classford, was also on hand to welcome us and help us settle in Canada. The feeling was nothing I had ever experienced before: the joy of being reunited, together again, but with new sights in a totally different place. I had never seen so many white people. The size of the airport, the size of everything made my heart pound and my eyes wander. But I was not used to the quiet way people went about their business. The absence of laughter and loud voices seemed strange. I was thrilled and nervous at the same time.

As I entered my mother's apartment for the first time, something caught my eye and I stared in wonderment. There before me was a colour television set. It was Hockey Night in Canada. I remember watching and being mesmerized: the ice, long sticks, and players in their padded gear. But most of all, it was their speed. It was dazzling.

Later, I learned the name of one of the teams, the Montréal Canadiens. Of course, Toronto's team is the Maple Leafs, who I am still hoping will bring the Stanley Cup home again. But when I arrived in Toronto in April 1976, I was first introduced to hockey by watching the Canadiens and the Boston Bruins.

Although the game of hockey was completely new to me, the skill of Guy Lafleur, Mario Tremblay, Ken Dryden and others was clearly evident. It was the NHL playoffs. I could tell from all the attention that hockey was a great and highly competitive sport. In addition to my own excitement of finally being in Canada and the joy of a full-blown reunion with my mother about to happen, the game on television caught my eye. Little did I realize, in a few months there would be another sporting event which would absorb me in a way that would mark my future... the Montréal Olympic Games.

Some would say it was a coincidence that I came to Canada in the same year as the Montréal Games. But I do not think so. Did my mother plan it that way? She would say it was God's Will. Looking back now, I can see that everything took place just as it was meant to.

Because of my fond memories of the 1976 Montréal Games, I rank them as one of the best shows of sprinting talent ever. For me, it was a moment that added a fuel to my running career. Donald Quarrie of Jamaica, an athlete who had ignited my own inspiration to run, was matched up with Haseley Crawford of Trinidad and Tobago. They squared off and competed in what was to be an unforgettable head-to-head showdown, one the world had never seen. At least, I had never seen such a thing before.

I was approaching 15 years of age, 12 years before Seoul. Back in Jamaica, sports was like ackee and salt fish, the national dish. You ate it, drank it, and breathed it. And, if you could, you tried to relive the moments through your imagination. Lots of times my friends and I in Falmouth would imagine ourselves as sprinters, running barefoot on dirt tracks, laughing and having a great time as we pumped our arms and ran furiously. We were all Donald Quarries.

Yes, where I came from, sport was a big thing. Whether it was a cricket test match or the FIFA World Cup, everywhere there would be excited talk with people glued to their black and white television set, if they had one, or their ears tuned in to a radio. It was not unusual to see someone riding a bicycle and holding a transistor radio, listening in while pedaling by. Whether at work or not, employed or not, this was one event holding us all in common, rich or poor, beggar man or thief. In Jamaica, the love for sports was raw, unfiltered and undiluted. It was pure unadulterated passion.

During the year of the Montréal Games, before I arrived in Toronto, I remember the hum was everywhere in Jamaica... in the homes, bars and shops, in the fields, streets and markets, and even in the banks and schools. Men, women and children followed the pre-Olympic reports as they worked or played, huddling together to follow the drama, anxiously waiting to see it unfold. This was the Jamaica I knew. And now that I was in Toronto, it wasn't any different. The phone kept ringing with friends and family asking for updates. They would ask with pride as if we all personally knew Quarrie and Crawford.

Quarrie in particular was a local hero. He was loved and admired unconditionally. Quarrie could do no wrong. We lived and died with him. His success was ours, and his failures, too. Even if he did not win or do well, we still embraced him. He was still our hero, no matter what. He was 25 at that time, in the prime of his sprinting career. He had performed consistently well. In 1976, Jamaican hopes and dreams were riding on his shoulders and his speed. This bond between athlete and country was not lost on me. It was like a bond between members of a family and it was special.

When Quarrie ran, the Island would practically shut down to witness the showdown. Now that I was in Canada, this had not changed. I was not going to miss it. I asked my sister if we could go to Montréal to see the Games. "No," she said and then explained, "Too far, too expensive." I cried. I wanted to go so badly. "You can watch it on TV," she tried to console me.

The Montréal Games were truly special for many reasons. There were controversial boycotts, one of them concerning South African apartheid. A lot of African countries, as well as Guyana, chose not to participate. Jamaica was anti-apartheid but was more pro-Quarrie. To keep Quarrie from running would have created a real national crisis. Sports and politics, even back then, ran in lanes one and two.

Aside from the politics, it was the intensity of athletic competition that made the Montréal Games exciting. Athletic performance rose to a new level. A 14-year-old girl about the same age as me, Nadia Comaneci of Romania, became the first gymnast to score perfect tens a crazy seven times, winning three gold medals. She certainly raised the bar. Bruce Jenner of the USA also set a world record in the decathlon to earn a place on Wheaties cereal boxes and other endorsements.

In the pool, American men ruled, as did the German women. The German female team won all but two gold medals. Later, there were suspicions about their illegal use of injected testosterone. Allegations about illegal use of performance-enhancing substances did not start with me and would not end with me either.

In weightlifting, Vasiliy Alexseyev, a Russian super heavyweight, asserted himself over his German competitors to win one of the seven gold medals won by the Soviet Union that year. And in boxing, the Spinks brothers, Michael and Leon, took home gold to their families and for the USA. And then there was Ray Leonard, with a picture of his girlfriend and baby taped to his socks, boxing his way skillfully into Olympic history as a mesmerizing light welterweight. Sugar Ray, indeed.

Not to be outdone, Cuba, Jamaica's neighbor to the north, shone, too. Teofilo Stevenson, considered to be one of the greatest Olympic boxers, had no match as a heavyweight. Cuba picked up 13 medals that year, including six gold. Many Jamaicans regarded Alberto Juantorena with great respect. He won two gold medals in the 400 and 800 metres. Had he been Jamaican, he would have been right up there with Quarrie in my opinion.

Canada as the host country did not win a single gold medal at the Montréal Summer Olympics. Winning five silver and six bronze, Canada was the first and only host country that did not win gold at the Summer Games. Right then and there, I felt I needed to do something in a positive way to change this. My dream was born: I was motivated to go out and win a gold medal for Canada. Of course, at the Vancouver 2010 Games, I'm proud to note that Canada more than made up for it by winning the most gold medals won by any country at a single Winter Olympics.

Despite Canada not winning gold in Montréal, the Games were special because of the level of strong competition and the strength of the athletes' performances. The Montréal Games were especially important to me because of Donald Quarrie, the man we called DQ. It was all about the sprints and DQ had those locked up. But first he had to get by the Trinidadian Crawford in the 100 metres. The race was on. I remember heated debates about who was faster, Quarrie or Crawford. We were, of course, partial to Quarrie. But Crawford was big and powerful and had won some world-class races. He had beaten DQ in the semifinals for the 100 metres. But the way we saw it, Quarrie was saving his strength and there was no way he was about to lose in the finals. As far as we were concerned, the 100 and 200 belonged to DQ, no discussion.

DQ was for us more than just a sprinter or an athlete. He had become our hero. Politically and socially, Quarrie represented an ideal, like Jesse Owens. Jesse Owens was celebrated for the four gold medals he won at the 1936 Berlin Olympics, defying the odds to become known as one of the greatest athletes of the 20th century. But for lovers of track and field, it was his dominant performance on the track and in the long jump that made Jesse Owens renowned.

To be a multiple Olympic gold medalist is truly amazing. People without the experience really have no idea how much it takes to be the best in the world in any one sport. To be the best in four different events is mystifying. I do acknowledge the achievement of Carl Lewis who won four gold medals in the 1984 Los Angeles Games. I was happy for him and impressed by his performance. Donald Quarrie was like that too... someone really and truly special. Before Quarrie, there was Arthur Wint, Herb McKenley and George Rhoden, Jamaica's celebrated Olympic heroes from a previous generation.

But for my generation, it was DQ's time. In 1976, we expected to see his greatness confirmed on top of the Olympic podium, not once but twice, with a champion's wreath and gold medals around his neck, the sound of the Jamaican anthem playing gloriously. We expected him to get a hero's welcome when he returned home. We were ready to give him a coronation, to crown him the king of sprints. I was giddy and euphoric as a young teen watching this epic athletic drama unfold. The race had not even been run yet, much less won. My brother and I were beside ourselves with anticipation.

Quarrie, of course, was no stranger to set backs. All athletes face them from time to time and he had his fair share. He competed in four Olympic Games. In 1968, at age 17, he was injured during training and could not compete. In 1972, he again was injured at the Munich Games. He attempted the 200 metre race but later withdrew due to a pulled muscle. In 1976, everyone waited with anticipation to see if DQ would be healthy. When news came that he was in tip-top shape, expectations soared. Later in 1980, he was coming off a serious car crash when he competed in the Moscow Games and still he grabbed a bronze at those Games in the 200 metre. In 1984, he ran in the 4 x 100 metre relay.

In total, Donald Quarrie won four Olympic medals, one gold, two silver and one bronze. He was also victorious in the Commonwealth and Pan American Games. My admiration for him, and what he was able to do despite the adversity he faced, cannot be overstated. He ran the 100 metre, 200 metre and a leg in the 4 x 100 metre relay for Jamaica as if it was nothing. He was durable and placed himself among the likes of others such as Tommy Smith whose record he equaled in the 200 metre during the Pan

American Games in South America in 1971. Donald Quarrie was a very important role model for me, someone I looked up to for inspiration. Surprisingly, Bryan revealed to me through his spiritual gift of discernment that Donald Quarrie never looked at himself as a hero or icon, but as a simple man who got a lucky break.

History records Donald Quarrie lost the 100 metre to the powerful Haseley Crawford in the 1976 Games. Crawford, sporting a pair of yellow running spikes to go with the Trinidadian colours of red, black and white, hit a gear and thrust his body across the finish line, so agonizingly close, to take the gold from us. It was unbelievable: 10.06 and 10.07. My, my, that was close! Crawford was a worthy competitor. He was powerful and could convert that power into speed. At over six feet tall, he was intimidating but not to DQ. As far as Jamaicans were concerned, Quarrie was still the faster of the two. After all, he had been leading the race until that decisive moment.

So we waited. There was still the 200 metre race. It was July 26, 1976, come back time. Quarrie was out of the blocks with lightening speed. Running out of lane two, he had already gained ground after his opening strides. No one ran the curve like DQ and on this day he was vintage. Then something strange happened. Crawford was running in lane five. As if suddenly seeing DQ pulling closer and sensing competitive pressure, Crawford stalled and pulled up and out of the race. DQ then seemed to have lost some of his momentum as the other competitors began to win back some ground down the stretch.

Man, talk about nerves! The noise of us cheering Quarrie on must have carried all the way to Montréal, pushing him to hold off the challenge that was closing in fast. We yelled louder. Another defeat was impossible. Silver was not good enough. As if Quarrie heard us, he accelerated and held his surge, holding off his rivals, showing his experience to win the race in 20.22 seconds. And we yelled even louder now, jumping and slapping hands as if we always knew. And that is how it started for me, this dream of becoming an Olympic sprinter.

Two years later in 1978, Dezrine and Clare joined us in Canada. My father visited Toronto a number of times as well but did not emigrate. He felt he needed to attend to his business in Jamaica. He loved the water and he loved the slower lifestyle back home. He knew that Canada was a beautiful country, but his heart was really in Jamaica. So, my father chose to stay there, maintain the family home, and provide support for his family the best way he could, albeit from afar. He visited us in Canada as often as possible.

My parents remained married until my father's death in 1990. Despite the distance between Jamaica and Canada, they successfully managed to raise their children together. Our family was one of the few we knew that had two parents. We always knew they both loved us, regardless of the distance separating us. However, the transition for the children was difficult: We had moved from a large family home with a couple of acres of land and lush gardens in Jamaica to a three bedroom apartment in a big city.

I tried to pretend I was still in Falmouth with my friends. But rather than swim at the beach, or roam freely about without care, I would play down by the creek near our apartment with my new friends in Canada. We would hunt birds, pick crab apples, try to catch fish and generally just be boys, as if we were still in the Caribbean.

One day, one of my friends aimed and pulled his slingshot at a pigeon. He hit and killed the bird. It was lunchtime. So, he took the pigeon to a secluded spot, started a fire and proceeded to pluck and cook it. In Jamaica we had a name for this kind of rough outdoor cooking. When someone said he was going to "run a boat," he meant he was going to perform the culinary version of the television program, Survivor: cook on an open fire with provisions rustled up at short notice, taking contributions from whomever would partake. Usually, it was a one-pot meal intended to feed everyone present. If the meal was a success, the boat was said to have landed safely. If, on the other hand, there was some misfortune that led to a disaster, the boat was said to have run aground.

He never had a chance to launch his boat with the pigeon that day. Worse than running aground, he was shipwrecked before he began. Not too long after he started, the police showed up, telling us he could get in a lot of trouble for this. We were so afraid. My friend immediately threw away the bird, quickly extinguished the fire with his feet and ran away. That day, I learned Toronto was very different from Jamaica. I immediately realized this was uncivilized behaviour and disrespectful to animals. Today, through one of my sessions with Bryan, I have asked God to forgive me for playing any role in causing the death of that bird. And I was glad to get this off my shoulders.

The pigeon episode was one of many culture shocks I experienced during my first year in Toronto. Another was the long Canadian winter. The postcards my mother used to send us did not prepare me for the reality of winter. Boots, scarf and a hat along with layered clothing were all too much for me. I was not used to it. A shirt, sweater and pants were all I had ever worn before.

My first experience with frostbite was very painful. But, I was more worried for my mother. She never complained but I could clearly see she suffered from the cold. She had broken her ankle in a car accident and it would swell up from time to time. The cold probably did not help. I would ask her about it. I am sure she ached. But before I could express any concern, she would hurriedly put on her boots and head out the door yelling, "Ben, don't worry about it." I would stare at her through the window, not taking my eyes off her until she disappeared down the road.

Cars would come and go. Like many young boys, I loved cars and saw them as a symbol of achievement. I would often dream about the day I would own a luxury car and wondered how I would achieve such success. I would dream of one day owning one so my mother would never be frostbitten again. And if I was successful, nor would I.

When I was not looking out the window and dreaming of fancy cars, I would watch television or listen to music. I continued my love of movies, particularly westerns, but now they were available to me on television in Canada! My favourite TV show was Sanford and Son. I can honestly say that I have watched every episode several times, and regularly recite many of the lines. In fact, I still often relate real life situations to some of those I watched on the shows, reeling off many of Fred Sanford's comments and jokes.

I had a very difficult time fitting into my new school. Pierre LaPorte Public School was located in a low-income area of Toronto, not exactly the slums, but close. I felt reserved and uncertain there. I remained quiet in class, not saying much, trying to deal with my misgivings in silence. I preferred to wait for the right time and the right place to speak: This school did not seem like the right place to me.

I was really shy and quite small for my age. Weighing only 93 pounds, I was a target for the school bullies. One day, I was approached by one of my tormentors and his buddy. Trying to establish their superiority, he and his friend challenged me to a race. They may have heard of my reputation as a runner; I don't know. If they did, they must have thought they could beat me and prove their dominance. For me, it was a chance to run for my freedom, freedom from harassment and intimidation.

I accepted their challenge but with a wager: If I won, no more bullying and name calling. They agreed. The race was on. I remember as if it were yesterday, word spreading across the school like wild fire. I was nobody but everyone knew these boys. They had the reputation of being highly competitive. The stakes were high. There was no backing down.

Half past noon was showdown. Lunch in the cafeteria was quick that day, as everyone headed outside to witness the spectacle. The teachers on duty in the cafeteria could not help but notice this rapid exodus, triggering an alarm that a schoolyard brawl was about to break out. By then, the tension had escalated. The teachers called the principal and everyone headed out, teachers and all, to the track where an agitated crowd quickly gathered. The boys showed up with their girlfriends, ready to show off and claim bragging rights. I remember the teachers looking on, stunned by the sight of a student-organized event. Open-mouthed, they watched as a student with a bullhorn gave the countdown and signaled the start of the race.

My speed was not jaw-dropping but I won that day. It was a big victory. I won by a full stride. The crowd of students swirled with mixed emotions. Many of them swarmed me. Some wanted to congratulate me. Some expressed their disappointment to me. I ended my days of being bullied but still, I felt badly for the kid I beat. My father taught me that when I win in life, I should not go bragging about it. It's better to be silent, and through thought, express and have compassion to the one who lost. My performance that day caught the attention of the physical education teacher. Shortly after that race, I was asked to join my school's track and field team.

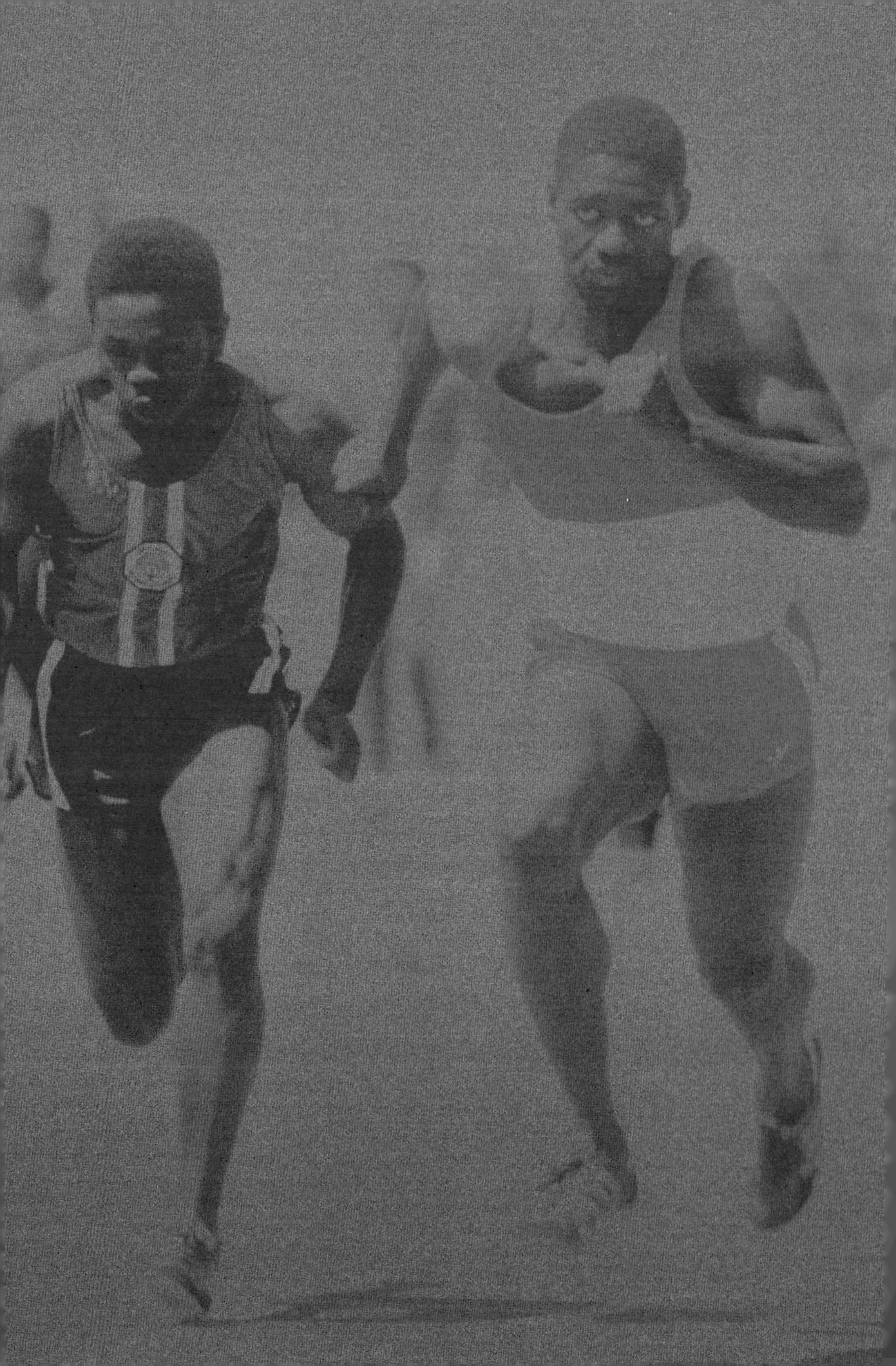

CHAPTER 8

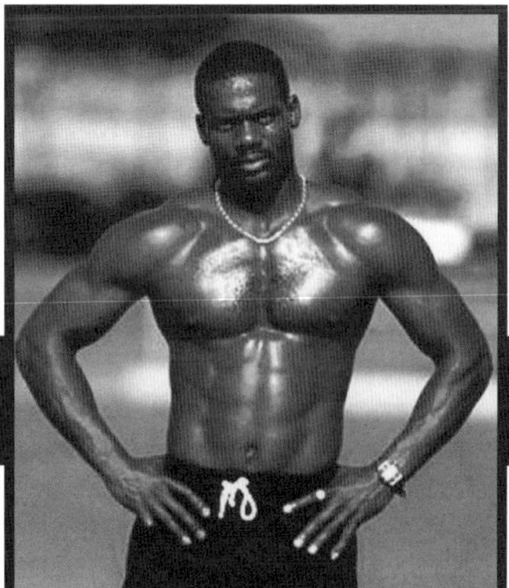

Training

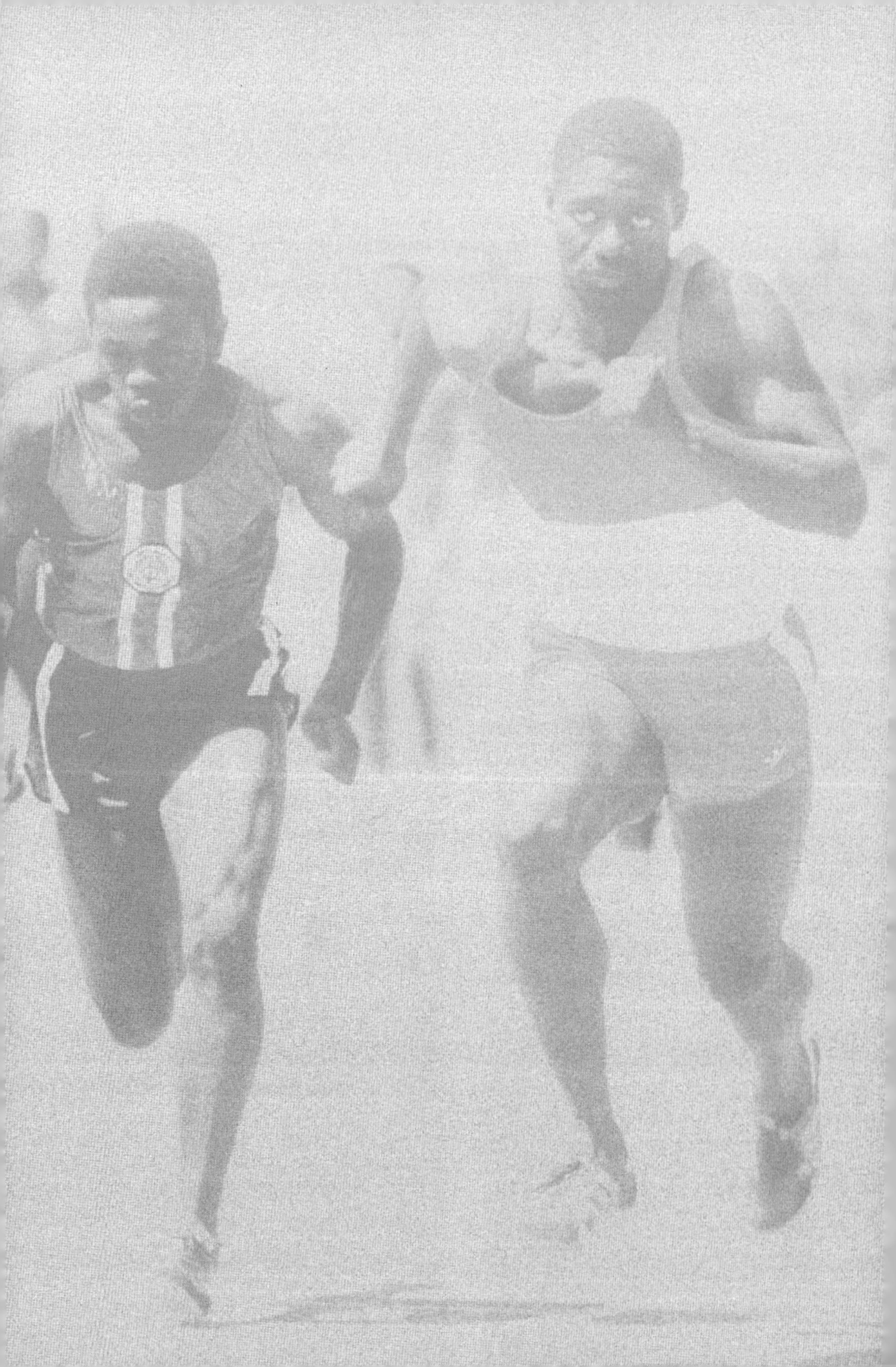

CHAPTER 8

Training

In high school, I started to take track and field more seriously than I ever had before. My older brother, Edward, was working toward a track scholarship. He asked me about two ribbons I had brought home from school. "Where did these come from?" he inquired. I was thrilled that he was interested. I told him I had won them and invited him to watch me compete. A week later, he told me to come with him to his track club, the Scarborough Optimists, to meet his coach, Charlie Francis. I did not have any gear but he said, "No matter, come anyway."

I was happy for the success Edward experienced at his track events. However, a part of me knew if I were to do better than him, on some level, the closeness of our relationship might be compromised at times. The family connection was very important to me. And on some level, winning became even more important, because I intuitively knew I had responsibility to help family members who were not as fortunate as me. I went through some tough lessons about being able to give to others unconditionally, particularly when I knew not everyone I helped truly appreciated my help. And this was not always easy for me.

I wanted to ask God what money meant to me in the early part of my career.

Ben, I brought you into this life for you to be able to experience your true self, for you to eventually achieve inner peace, knowing quite well that money would not drive you to achieve many goals in your life. Yes, you lost a great opportunity in this life... for many who have gone through your experience would have by now taken their own life... because money became their god, became their blanket, and became their security. But money failed to give them inner peace and always kept them on a journey of unfulfillment. I made you strong. I made you know, through all the ups and downs you would go through, there would be times you went away from Me. But it was always destined for you to come back to Me. Money is a curse for many. Money is a destructive force for great nations. But only through time, all shall return to Me, only to find the true inner peace is with Me.

My family and my spiritual connection to God gave me the inner strength to not give up and always work hard to achieve whatever goal presented itself to me. And I am so glad my brother was there for me. Having a big brother was a blessing. Had it not been for him, I may not have been able to connect with my destiny as quickly as I did. He knew of my growing boredom and how I missed my friends and the ocean in Falmouth. He must have seen me becoming swallowed up by this new big city, not knowing where to go or what to do. He knew I had the desire to run. But most of all, he saw I needed something constructive to occupy my time: I needed to fight off idleness and the temptations of the streets. I am very thankful my brother cared enough to mentor me. I am grateful to my brother for contributing to my early beginnings as a sprinter.

I asked Bryan about my boredom. The Lord set the record straight:

Ben, you're asking Me to provide you with an explanation about the boredom you believe you had, just being new to Canada. Your boredom, at times, got confused with many different influences in your life. Your boredom had nothing to do with the fact that you were in Canada, away from Jamaica. You have only experienced boredom throughout your life when you are not running or when you are not training. This is the only time that you have experienced boredom. Ben, you came into this world to be a sprinter and to run for the Heavens.

I responded, "Oh that makes sense." I can see now I was simply searching for my life's purpose. I was made to run. That is why I have a unique start. Nobody duplicated it. Moving to Toronto was not the problem. The problem was just being in a time of transition and the uncertainty of my teen years.

I joined the Scarborough Optimist Track Club in 1977, a privately funded club organized by Mr. Ross Earl, a physical education teacher at a Scarborough public school. Mr. Earl hired Charlie Francis as coach. Charlie had represented Canada in the Munich Olympic Games in 1972 and was the Canadian 100 metre champion in 1970, 1971, and 1973.

Charlie had gained most of his formal training through a track scholarship to Stanford University. From personal experience, he was well acquainted with the fact that, historically, there had been no organized track program in Canada. He thought Canadian sprinting needed more recognition from sport administrators. So when his sprinting career ended abruptly, he was keen to pass on the benefit of his knowledge. We greatly improved with his instruction.

In 1978, I participated in the trials for the Commonwealth Games to be held in Edmonton that year. I was one of the top juniors in Canada at the time. I was sure I had finished fourth in the semi to move on to the final, the race which would determine who would represent Canada in Edmonton. However, the finish times were not posted. I asked an official which lane I would be in for the final. They informed me I had come in fifth and did not make the final. But I thought I came in fourth and I was very disappointed.

I took my bag with all of my gear, went off by myself away from my teammates and cried. Even though I had only been training for a year, I was already among the top runners in Canada. But I believed the Canadian sports body did not recognize my accomplishments because of Charlie's poor relationship with the Canadian Track and Field

Association (CTFA). They did not card me as a Canadian athlete, an official status which would have provided me with some financial assistance. To me, this felt deliberate. I thought the treatment I received was very discouraging. It was as if they wanted me to quit. I did not feel like I was being supported.

I asked Bryan about this perceived mistake. Why did they tell me I came in fifth, when I was really fourth? Again, God set the record straight for me:

Ben, for what you experienced by coming in fifth was designed for you to work even harder. For even at that time, you could have done more. You had many expectations, and through these expectations, you were disappointed. But you must remember: It is I Who delivers the fruits of life to you. It is I Who knows when you are ready. At that time, you were not ready. At that time, you had not proven yourself. For coming in fifth only made you work harder to eventually become number one.

In Edmonton, and even to this date, many Olympians have a subconscious fear of winning over the United States of America. Even back in the time of your Edmonton trials, the Canadian government had a subconscious fear of winning over the United States. I say to you, Ben, and to all My Children: Where there is complete Truth, there is no fear. Had things been different, you would have received your financial support.

I was surprised to learn that I really had placed fifth. The officials were right after all. It's amazing how God even set that up, so I would try that much harder. It worked! Even at the time, after I had recovered from my disappointment, I consoled myself by knowing sooner or later I would be able to prove myself to the Canadian sports bodies.

The Scarborough Optimist Club participated in a meet in the upscale Lawrence Park neighbourhood of Toronto every year. This was a private track meet organized and funded by Mr. Percy Duncan. Percy himself was involved in track as a young boy in British Guyana. He would later go on to become my coach in 1991 and 1992. At this meet in 1979, our Club was finally noticed for its achievements. At one time, a representative of

Athletics Canada had told Ross Earl the only reason the Scarborough Optimist Club had great athletes was because the boat from Jamaica stopped in Toronto: It had nothing to do with coaching ability.

I asked Bryan to ask the Lord, why is it that Jamaicans hold a high standard in sprinting?

Ben, so you ask Me, why do many Jamaicans have such high standards for sprinting? I will answer the question this way: It is not about one being better than the other. It is not about one being superior over another. It is about these sprinters, who come from Jamaica, bringing hope to the people of Jamaica who have suffered, who have gone, in many cases, unrecognized. I will use My Children in various ways to bring joy to those who suffer. For the sprinters that have come from Jamaica have brought joy and hope to many. For I love all My Children, regardless of what race they are. For one ethnic race cannot exist without all others. This is part of the Math Equation of God.

Thank You, Father. I am hoping Usain Bolt will receive and process this Truth. I would love to see Usain recognize and accept that God made him a runner from the day he was born... that a runner is born, not made. I pray he will take my life experience as an example and try to avoid the same pitfalls.

At the Black Heritage Track Meet at Lawrence Park Collegiate School in 1979, the Scarborough Optimist Club won every event! After the meet, Charlie Francis and Ross Earl were approached by the Canadian Federation and asked for the contact information for their athletes. Now the government was interested in funding the Club. It was a show of good faith on their part.

By 1980, I had arrived at a point where I thought I could compete at an Olympic standard. While I was not yet carded, I still pressed on in the hope that I would have an opportunity to prove myself. And then crushing news came: Canada joined the USA in boycotting the Moscow Games. The USA objected to the Russian invasion of Afghanistan.

Four years later when the Games were held in Los Angeles, the Russians replied with a boycott of their own. I never completely understood why politics had to interfere with our sport. So I asked Bryan if God would tell me, what does politics have to do with sports?

Ben, you ask the question, what does politics have to do with sports? Do you understand the question that you are asking? Should you not be asking the question: why is it that heads of states are not able to solve many of the problems among themselves, and between one leader and another? Many of these world leaders, through their own false beliefs, have become separated from Me. But on a conscious level, they truly believe that they are connected to Me, that I am endorsing conflict and I am endorsing war. For I only endorse unconditional love and unconditional forgiveness. Many leaders throughout history have taken on the role of God, having a distorted understanding of Who I am. And when they cause another to lose a limb, to lose their life, they have no compassion. They are not determined to stop the suffering. For many of these world leaders take it upon themselves to boycott Olympic events from a position of fear... fear that they will not do as well, that they will be number two.... or from a position of becoming the punishing god that I am not.

Wow, that's very strong. I was blown away hearing that.

The athletes caught between the politics had dedicated themselves, through very hard work, to becoming the best they could be, only to be told they would have to wait. Fortunately for me, I was still young and had time on my side. But there were others who would never have another chance to perform at their peak and at the same level. To have that moment slip by without even a chance to compete is one of the most hurtful things that can happen to an athlete. I cried after my setback at the Commonwealth Game trials, but for those athletes who were completely denied the chance to compete after building their hopes up so high, it must have been many times more devastating.

The Optimist Club did have great coaching. I was finally carded in fall 1980. Many of my fellow teammates from the Optimist Club competed in Rome at the World Championships in 1987 when I set the new world record. I felt very special being a part of this program along with these people. They were not only my teammates, but also my friends: Desai Williams, Mark McCoy, Angella Issajenko and Tony Sharpe. The Club also brought me into contact with the people who would later become part of my entourage, eventually supporting my Olympic efforts. These included Charlie Francis who was my coach; Ross Earl, my adviser; Jamie Astaphan, the team's doctor; Larry Heidebrecht, my agent; and Waldemar Matuszewski, my physio- and massage therapist. This may seem like a lot of people. But no world-class athlete gets to that level without vital support from numerous people. These individuals were a large part of my life leading up to Seoul.

Of course, one of the most important people to any athlete is his or her coach. When I first began training with Charlie at the Scarborough Optimist Track Club, I was not all that promising as an athlete. I could barely run one lap around the club track. Even other members of the club doubted my ability and said so. I recall one teammate saying to me, if I ever beat him, it would be time for him to retire. I responded by saying I had only just started my training, give me six months. His words inspired me to train harder and made me more determined to beat him. I eventually did... and he quit the team, just as he said he would.

When training outdoors became unbearable in the winter, we moved our activity elsewhere. Each training day, I would make the long trip to downtown Toronto by the shores of Lake Ontario to practice at the Canadian National Exhibition (CNE) where they had an indoor facility called the Swine Pavilion. We nicknamed it the Pig Palace. Every day after class, I would run for the bus, hop on the subway, and then take a streetcar to the Pig Palace. The lake was lovely but it was not my Jamaican sea. The beaches were not like the ones I knew. Nevertheless, I would race down to the lakeshore, not for swimming but rather to run and to train.

The Palace was disgusting. The air stunk from rubber track smell mixing with farm animals' odour from below. Even so, I stayed focused on my purpose and concentrated on the goals of my training. For the first time, I began to see myself as a runner and knew it was going to become my passion and my future. I could see so many possibilities and dreams within my grasp. But before I could attain my dreams, there would be obstacles to overcome.

While the Pig Palace was the place to train during the winter, we could only train there until March. The spring thaw was still too cold for outdoor training. Charlie suggested we go south so as not to lose any training time. These road trips were exciting to me as a teenager but my family and I could not afford the expenses. Charlie was generous: While the club paid for some of our travel costs, Charlie would often contribute his own money to help out. I enjoyed these outings, the jovial friendships with my teammates, the practical jokes we played on each other and the idle chatter. But I was always aware of how limited my means were and how dependent I was on others. Some of these trips took us to Tennessee and Florida. Other times, we went overseas to Europe. This exposure helped me to better understand what it would take to compete at an international level: sacrifice, hard work and determination.

Track and field training consists of drills repeated over and over again, programming and conditioning the mind and body to perform under the pressure of race conditions. It involves perfecting techniques designed for maximum explosive speed and acceleration, and applying proven and sometimes innovative methods. For this, Charlie was renowned. Timing was the most important thing in my line of running. Sprints are measured in seconds and fractions of a second. Every hundredth of a second counts. One one-hundredth of a second can make the difference between winning and losing. By 1979, I had become the Canadian 100 metre Junior Champion with a time of 10.60. I was 17 and getting ready to make a bid for international competition.

Depending on the season, I would spend up to forty hours per week training. It was a full-time job. The level of commitment required had to be nothing less. Each day after training, I would go home, eat, shower and go to bed exhausted. I would be so fatigued that sometimes I would fall asleep while eating supper, going directly to bed without even so much as a shower. The next day, I would be back at it again. We trained extremely hard.

Keeping up a social life was next to impossible with my busy training schedule. I had two sets of friends, my schoolmates and my track mates. But in truth, they were only acquaintances. I really did not have any close friends at all. After school, I would catch a bus to the training track. Going to the park to hang out with schoolmates was not an option for me. So I never really got close to any of my schoolmates, although I did try to keep in touch with a handful of them over the years. As for my track mates, I only saw them at the track. None of us had a car or much time or money to socialize. Off the track, we lived in different worlds. If anything, it was our road trips together that helped to strengthen our friendships.

Pursuing part-time employment was also not possible for me due to my demanding training schedule. I kept up school where I could but my life after 1977 revolved around training. Initially, it was my mother who financed my training. Sometimes she would work overtime to help with my expenses such as travel and other incidentals. By the end of 1980, I was receiving a small stipend every three months from the government as a carded athlete. But it was still a stretch trying to cover rent, food, clothing and other bills.

Charlie did what he could to help and sometimes went over and beyond his role as coach. For instance, he once sold his prized Aston Martin so as to finance our travel south to train during the unforgiving cold months. There were other times when he would put some of us up, as we struggled through our own individual difficulties.

As a contrast, our American counterparts were well supported financially and otherwise. It was always impressive to see their training facilities and to hear about their sophisticated training programs managed by well-paid coaches. I wonder what they would have thought of the Pig Palace. I asked Bryan to discern why I ended up with the Pig Palace and not the American Dream. God answered:

Ben, for what is the American Dream? For all those who hold dear to their heart the American Dream, do they hold Me close to their heart? Would you have done as well if I gave you the American Dream? The answer is no. I made you struggle, I made you become determined, much more determined, for you to understand that you did not need money to make you a winner. You just needed Me. You did not need anything else. For those who hold dear to their hearts the American Dream, did they make it because of Me?

These words warmed my heart. Back in those days, we just worked with what we had and made the best of it. The Lord's Words reminded me of what Charlie used to say, "If it's not broke, don't fix it."

I trained hard. But it was important not to stress the body and overwork the nervous system. The goal was to build endurance, stay fit and strong. On different days, we would focus on different aspects but recovery was extremely important. The key was to build, not to breakdown; to do high-intensity low-volume workouts.

Under Charlie's care and guidance, I gained weight and strength as my body matured from a teen-aged boy to a full-grown man. In 1978, I came in second in the 50 metres at the Canadian National Indoor Track and Field Championships. In 1980, I came in third in the 100 metres in the Canadian Men's Championships. I continued to improve and win championships over the next four years on the track and field circuit.

The more I trained, the more I began to understand the importance of working hard to perfect my technique and master my form. My competitive drive did not allow me to do any less. Eventually, I realized what worked for me and what did not. Sometimes this meant going back to the drawing board to adjust a few things. It was a process of trial and error.

One thing that became clear to me, for example, was the importance of upper body strength. That is why in 1980 I started working with weights. No one understood, at first, the value of what I was doing. But I could feel and see the results. Working out with weights helped me to train longer because I was stronger. Even Charlie, who had been slow to acknowledge the value of my approach, began to appreciate the overall results.

To me, it was important to understand my body. After all, my body was mine alone. I was the one living in it. Over time, I truly came to feel like my body was a well-oiled machine and I was the mechanic. I could tell immediately when and if something was not working properly or if there was a problem. When things were all lined up, I felt like a finely tuned Ferrari.

A key element to my success was my start. I developed a unique way of leaping out of the blocks with an explosive drive, propelling myself forward down the track ahead of my rivals. Through practice, I learned how to relax and, at the same time, keep enough tension to allow me to rip out of the starting blocks. After a while, it became natural to me. My start was so important to my performance. Most of my energy would be spent just getting out. I would then accelerate and hold that pace through to the end of the course. To beat me, my challenger would have to come from behind to catch and pass me. The trick was to maintain the speed to the finish, to last longer. And to last longer, I had to work on my endurance. It was a simple formula. The more I could maintain my initial pace, the faster my times would become.

During the early eighties, others began to recognize my potential. The York University Track and Field Centre had opened around this time, providing a home ground for us to train on all year round. Charlie, officially appointed as coach at the center, could now steadily work at grooming us for elite competitions. The Optimist Club formed the core of the sprinters and the club continued to pay most of the bills, covering our training camps, tours and equipment.

I was 19 when I ran in the World Cup trials in Venezuela in the summer of 1981. Some believe this race marked my arrival at the elite level. Although I placed second, my time of 10.25 seconds in the 100 metres was the fastest recorded time ever by a Canadian my age. Later that year, I began to excel over my teammates. Up until this time, they would beat me and carry the promise of victory. But now it was me who began to show signs of triumph. This raised eyebrows. When I became the first Canadian to reach the finals in three of Europe's most competitive meets, Cologne, Berlin and Zürich, many in the sport started to take notice. And while I did not place in the finals of these events, it was obvious that I had the potential to improve even more.

Later in 1981, another one of my dreams also came true in the World Cup held in Rome. I ran the anchor leg in the 4 x 100 metres relay, representing the Americas. The baton was handed to me by my longtime hero, Jamaica's Donald Quarrie. I ran to make him proud. To my surprise, the man I had looked up to in the 1976 Olympics embraced me as a young sprinter, offering me pointers and helping me now and again.

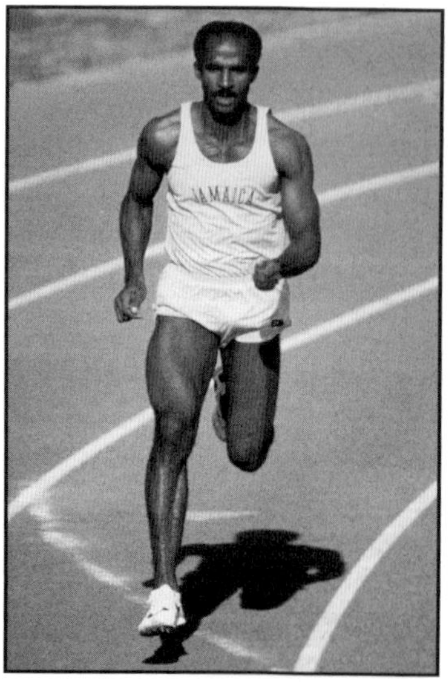

In 1981, the international limelight was on someone else, not me. The first time I raced against him was in Sudbury at the Pan American Juniors in 1980. He handily won the race in a time of 10.43, while I placed sixth at 10.88 seconds. Clearly, he was the faster man. He went on to become the crowned king of speed the following year, establishing himself as a household name. Track and Field News ranked him number one athlete of the year in 1982, 1983, and 1984. His name: Carl Lewis. Looking back today, I can see that a huge rivalry existed between Carl and me. I now recognize that this rivalry was a major contributing factor for me going through the experience of losing my gold medal in Seoul, on so many different levels.

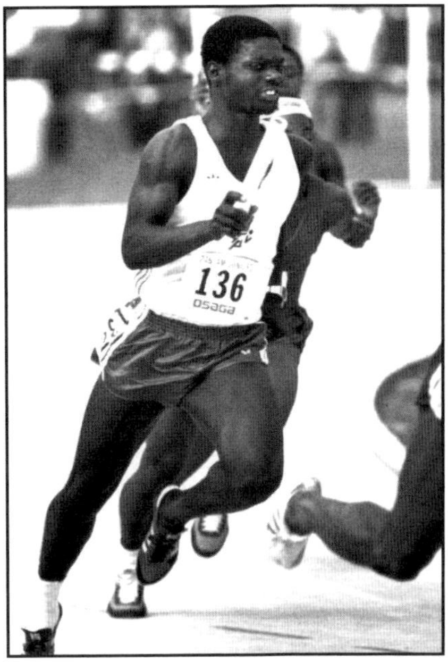

In the early 1980s, steroids became part of my training protocol. My mistake, as Bryan confirmed, was succumbing to the lure, the false belief that I needed a steroid protocol to level the playing field and keep up with the rivalry. In addition, if the science of steroids was correctly understood, everyone would know steroids do not make athletes run faster. Steroids only help the body with recovery, and only for the short-term.

Back in the early eighties, Carl Lewis was not concerned with me, not yet anyway. I knew it was only a matter of time before my work would pay off. Already my trademark speed out of the blocks was becoming standard. Those who knew me understood I did not cave under pressure. I knew my day would come. I told myself all I needed to do was keep working, keep improving and I would close the gap. I was not discouraged. I knew how to compete and I was not afraid.

I knew track and field was all there was for me. I gave up any thought of going to college or furthering my education, despite my father's wishes. I will never forget the day I quit college. I walked into class and gave all my books to someone I had befriended who I knew could not afford to buy them on his own. I approached the teacher, shook his hand, said, "Thank you very much," and left the school. This was a very serious decision for me. I realized once I left school behind, I was not going to turn back. I knew my father would be disappointed. Regardless, my mind was made up. Track and field would now become my means of earning my living on a full-time basis. There was no looking back.

At the time, I still lived with my mother in our three-bedroom apartment. There were some intense financial strains on the family, especially before I was carded. But when I finally started contributing to the household income, albeit a small amount, I was proud. My mother saw the talent in me. She even took a second job to finance my travel to track meets in order to advance my career. I devoted hours and hours each day to training and practice and can say that my mother was a huge motivation. I wanted her to be so proud and know the faith and confidence she placed in me was well-founded. I also wanted to give her a wonderful life. She worked hard her entire life and deserved the best I could provide.

I also had to work hard at interacting with others as I was extremely shy and had a bit of a speech impediment. It is difficult to develop into a great athlete under the best of circumstances, but the other personal issues I had to overcome meant I had to work that much harder to be better than other athletes. I believe this gave me the strength to deal with the tremendous heartaches I would encounter down the road.

When I was at home and not travelling, I attended church with my mother regularly. On some level, this helped to lay the foundation for my faith which, I admit, I have struggled with throughout the many challenges I have experienced. Bryan confirmed this. But going deeper, he discerned the core reason for my struggle was because of the anger and blame I had toward God for my parents not being together. Bryan discerned that this, along with past life issues, is the reason I experienced symptoms of chronic depression since the age of 17. I discussed these symptoms with Bryan. The heaviness of my depression was deep. But since my healing in 2008, the spiritual shackles of depression have been completely removed from me through Bryan's spiritual gift. I am so grateful that God gave me a mother who taught me the importance of faith. I know now that my relationship with God was the anchor that allowed me to reclaim my life and encourage others. I asked Bryan to ask God, what impact did my depression have on my ability as a sprinter?

Ben, you ask Me, what impact did depression have on your ability as a sprinter? Many of My Children have depression, and there are different types of depression. Many of My Children come into this life, already born with depression. For they carry with them great sadness, great trauma from another life experience. In your case, if you did not have depression, your performance would have been profound to the world. Races would have been able to be won much easier, as you would have been able to run much faster. Depression impacts the whole body. It can weaken the immune system. It can cause a longer recovery time from injury. It can cause one to lack the motivation to win. For when you ran and you won, in many cases you overcame your depression with your fear of failing. It is the fear of failing you had that made you appear that you were mentally on top of the world... where the signs of your depression were not noticed. But you are now free of your depression. This is no longer part of you. This is your moment. This is your moment, Ben.

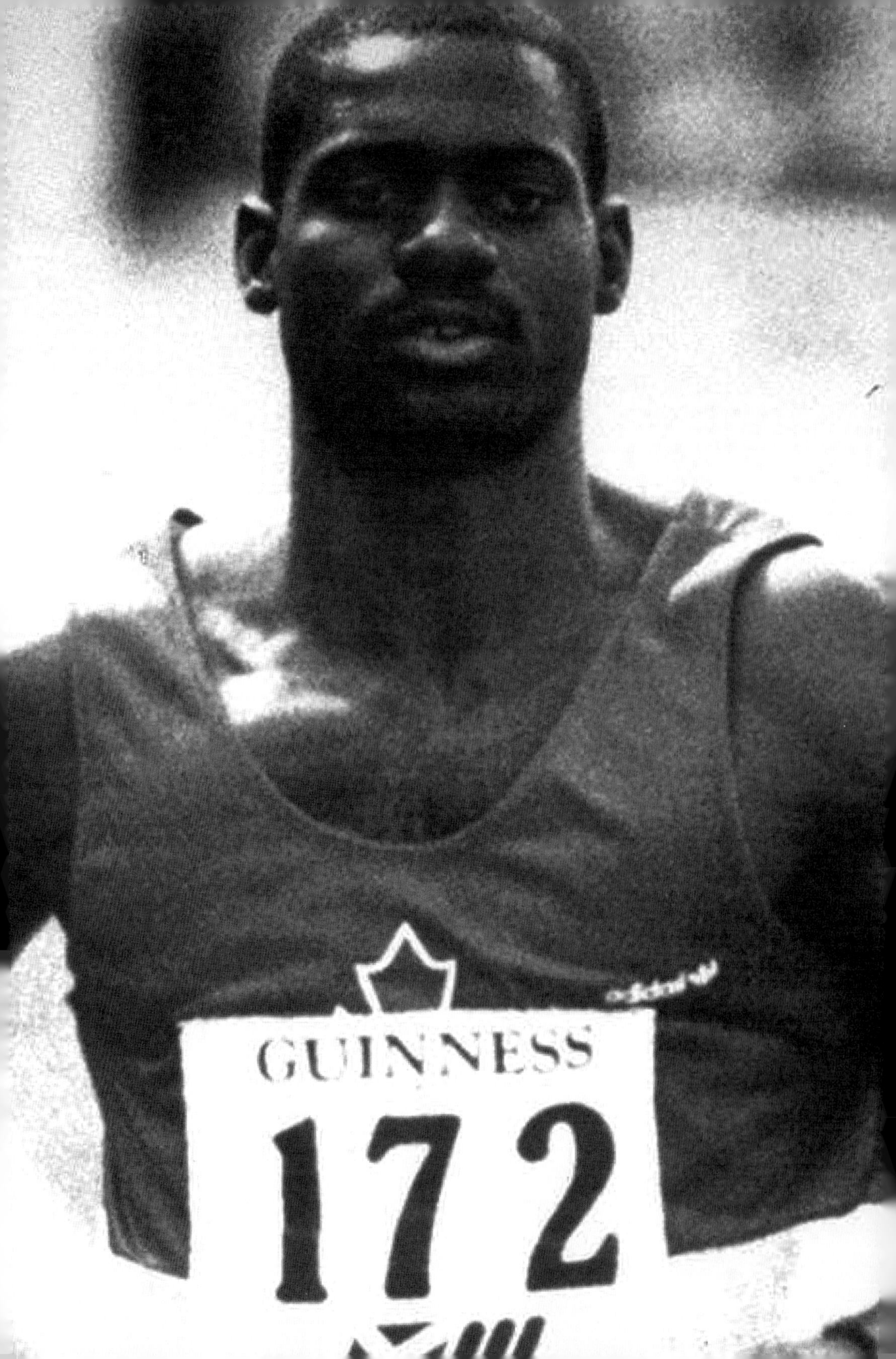
GUINNESS
172

CHAPTER 9

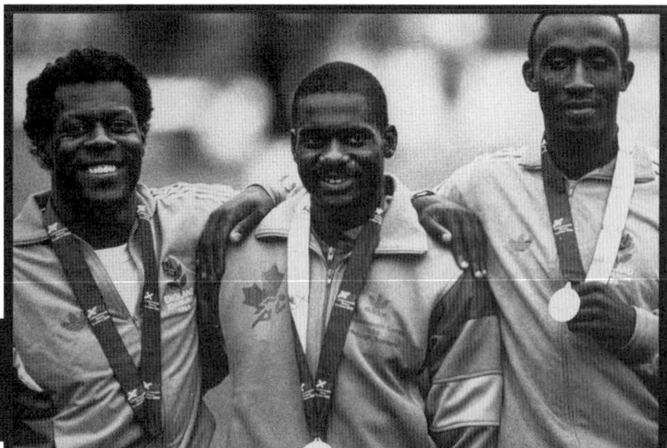

The Road to Rome

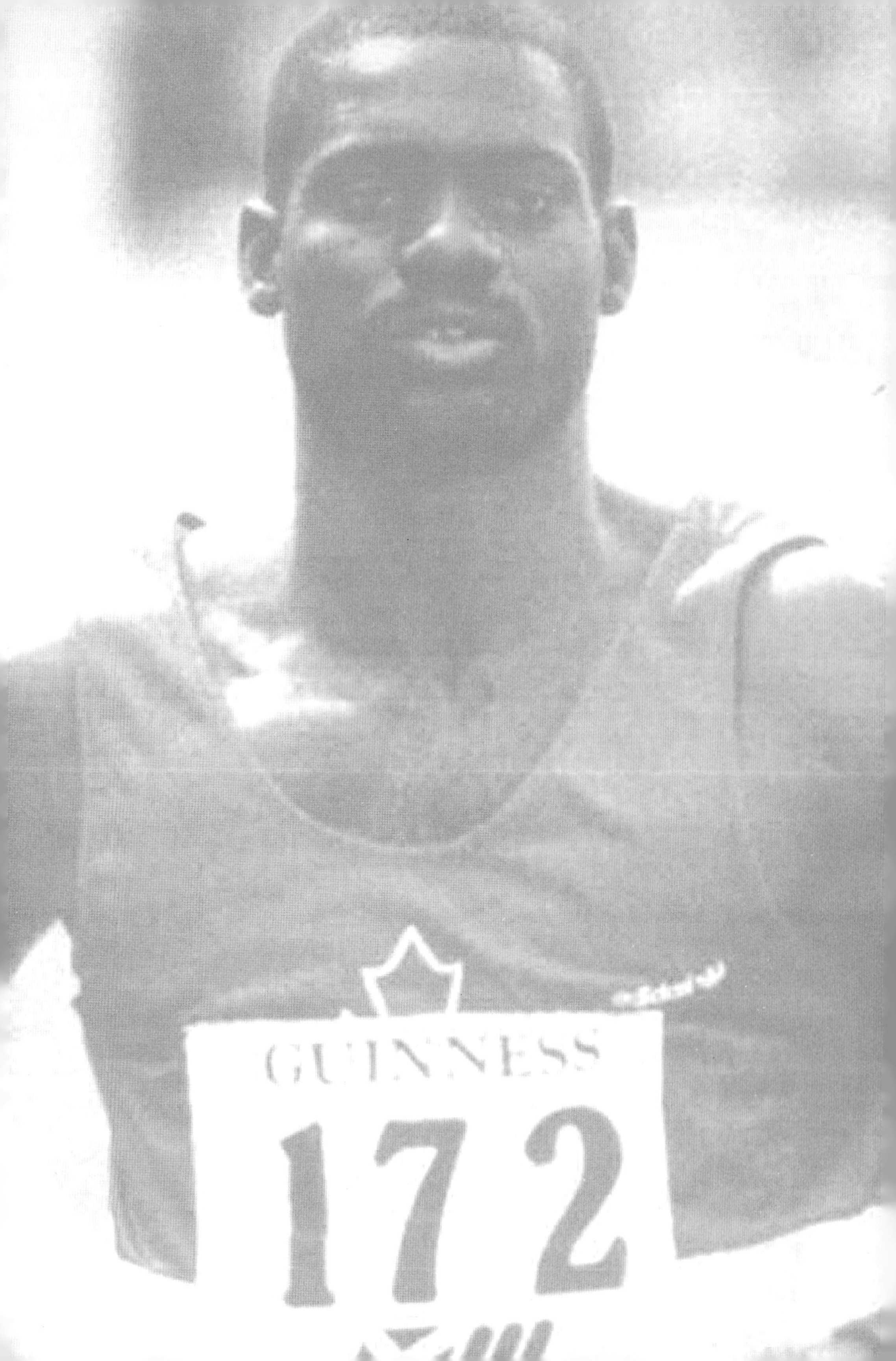
GUINNESS
172

CHAPTER 9

The Road to Rome

In 1980, nobody perceived me as a real contender to Carl Lewis. Although I was by then a top junior sprinter in Canada, I still did not have the profile to challenge him. But that would change.

At the 1982 Commonwealth Games held in Brisbane, Australia, our sprinters redeemed themselves after a dismal showing four years earlier. Angella won a gold and a bronze in the 100 and 200 metres respectively. The women's relay team picked up a gold in the 4 x 400 and a silver in the 4 x 100. Angella also ran in both of those relays, showing she was a true champion.

As for me, I won a silver medal in the 100 metres in Brisbane with a time of 10.05 seconds, wind-aided. I lost by three hundredths of a second to Allan Wells, considered at that time to be one of the best and already an Olympic champion. He caught me right at the finish. I could have held him off had I kept my form for just a bit longer. My showing in this race surprised everyone except me. I was coming off a knee injury and knew if I had been well, Wells would have been far behind. I was very proud of my achievement. At this point in my training, I knew I would be hard to beat over an 80 metre stretch.

When we sat down afterward to analyze the race, Charlie and I had a difference of opinion. He had not been pleased with my performance and criticized my hand position in the starting blocks. He argued I would have gained more ground coming out of the blocks had I adopted his approach. I, however, disagreed with his analysis, arguing that my start had nothing to do with my performance that day. Personally, I felt I had simply run out of steam at 90 metres. As far as I was concerned, it was my speed endurance that needed work, not my start.

Also about this time, my abilities began to be noticed internationally. By 1983, I had made significant progress. I had improved my personal best to 10.19 at an international meet held in Munich where I finished in first place.

I asked Bryan to discern why I came first in the Munich race. God told me what His Archives hold:

Ben, this race that you ask Me about... the question: why did you win the race? Ben, go back to that time. Go back to that time... how you had moments of giving up, and then racing, giving up, racing... but you always came back to the idea that you would continue to train, and that you would continue to race. For once again, it is the fear of failure that caused you to win.

While 10.19 was the best Canadian time ever in 1983, I was still not a challenge or a threat to Carl Lewis... at least, not yet. The 1983 World Championships in Helsinki provided my next opportunity to face him. But here again, he held sway. It was an American sweep. I came in twelfth. I was disappointed but not discouraged. I knew my subpar performance stemmed from a lack of consistent training over the summer when tendonitis in both knees hampered me. After the race I felt very bad. Charlie and I had a long talk afterward as we reviewed the race on tape. Donald Quarrie was there. That day, Donald told me I was the best starter in the world and I always came out in front. We all agreed: I had lost the race, not on the track, but in my mind.

I asked Bryan to discern why I came twelfth in the Helsinki race. The Lord said:

Ben, for I will give you a short answer to why you lost the race in Helsinki. Prior to the race, you had over trained and your body was tired. And you had a little bit of anger toward Charlie. And you were not focused on winning on that day. You did not have fear of failure to drive you. For many are not aware... 90% of those athletes who compete in the Olympics are mostly driven by fear of failure. Ben, you are not alone.

As I thought back to that time, I remembered Charlie wanted me to move my hands closer to the start line. I did not want to do it because I was more comfortable with my hands an inch and a half back. I forgive Charlie.

Meanwhile, Carl's career continued to soar. He pushed his time below 10 seconds that year. In Helsinki, he reaped gold in the long jump and the 4 x 100 relay. In 1983, he was superior to everyone else. While Carl was on top, I was more motivated to compete against him. He was definitely in a class by himself. I remember when I first saw him in Sudbury. I looked at him but he did not acknowledge me. He had this attitude of superiority about him as if he was the champ and I was the chump. I had a good laugh to myself about that.

Carl was, more than anything else, a major competitor. I regarded him as a force to be reckoned with, as Carl was a highly accomplished sprinter. Going into the 1984 Olympic Games in Los Angeles, I had the same outlook as always: I will simply try to do my best.

In addition to the fear of failure driving me to win, Bryan shared another interesting discernment with me about my race performance. He told me that whenever I had an expectation of beating Carl Lewis in a race, I would lose. The races I won, I won because I had no expectation of coming first. Looking back, I can see how this is true. The first few times I won against Carl Lewis were times I was tired or when my hotel reservations, or lack thereof, interfered with my preparations and I did not expect to win.

The 1984 Olympics experienced another boycott. This time, it was boycotted by the Soviets. These Games turned out to be a stage show for Lewis. On his home turf, fellow Americans came out to watch him perform his feats. And perform he did, winning four gold medals. I was considered an underdog, but I was not intimidated. I felt confident in my abilities.

Two months before the Games, I ran a wind-aided 10.01 at the Canadian Outdoor Championship. I felt I could have done even better, if conditions were right. Unfortunately, they were not. Held in Winnipeg, the Championships took place on a track insufficiently prepared for competition. Our training had not been optimal and our extensive traveling was hard on the body. We did not get the necessary down time to rest and recover. The schedule was just too hectic. Excuses aside, I was still prepared to run and win in Los Angeles. It was going to be my first Olympic Games and I was thrilled to be competing.

In LA, I was exposed to some of the negative aspects of staying in close proximity with other athletes. I roomed with Lennox Lewis in the Olympic Village. Lennox was a Canadian boxer originally from Great Britain. One day, I was playing pool in the lobby of the dorm and had the key to our room hanging around my neck. As I approached a shot, the key was dangling on the pool table so I took it from around my neck and placed it on a nearby chair. Lennox picked up the key and went out for about six hours leaving me stranded. When Lennox finally returned to the dorm much later, he found me waiting in the lobby. I approached him, asking why he left with the key and if he was going out why he didn't leave it at the front desk. Lennox told me I should not leave the key lying around.

Words were exchanged and then Lennox shoved me. I shoved him back. At the time, Lennox weighed approximately 230 lbs. to my 175 lbs. He grabbed me around my neck and started choking me. I was so strong I was able to lift him up off the ground and drop him on the pool table. The front desk staff called security and they came to break up the fight.

I asked Bryan about this incident. And he confirmed, through discernment, my fear of failure program came into play here. The fear of failure I had that motivated me to win races also motivated me when Lennox was choking me. The chemical reaction in my body took over and gave me that strength.

I spent the balance of my time in LA at a friend's house, nursing a sore neck and only went back to the village for my competitions. This incident with Lennox proved to be a distraction momentarily taking me away from my primary focus. I learned a valuable lesson that would help me in future competitions: I needed quite a bit of space to myself prior to races and I should not share that space with anyone else. I asked Bryan to confirm if this was the lesson that I learned from that experience. He discerned it was true.

I quickly realized my goal was to win, not just to compete. My renewed focus and determination took me through to the finals. Tony Sharpe made it through with me. Desai, who had left Charlie's team by then, did not make it. During the semifinals my hamstring started to act up. It was not injured but it was tight. I had a massage during the break before the finals and I felt fine.

Coming out of the blocks during the finals, I was called for a false start. I needed to be careful the next time around. I would be disqualified if I did it a second time. I took a deep breath knowing I had to hold back a little. The gun went off and I reacted slower than I normally would. With that, my advantage was gone. Normally ahead of the pack for the first 10 metres, I was trailing now, running fifth and far behind. Having faltered during my drive phase, I knew I had to make up for it with a surging acceleration. So, I gunned it.

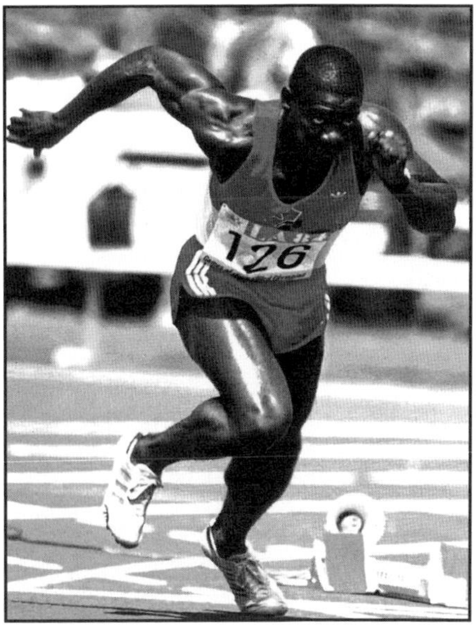

Halfway down, I had gained enough ground to overtake Carl Lewis and everyone else for the lead at 60 metres. This race was mine.

Or so I thought. Suddenly, my leg cramped up and I ran out of steam. I intended to use my lightening start to get out in front and then maintain to the finish, thereby taking the pressure off my hamstring. Unfortunately, that did not happen and I lost ground quickly. First, Lewis blew by, then Sam Graddy.

And that is how it ended, my first Olympic final. Lewis won the gold in 9.99. Graddy won silver in 10.19. I came away with the bronze medal with a time of 10.22. Could I have won? Of course I could have. I was not discouraged.

Carl won four gold medals at the 1984 Games. I acknowledge he is a great athlete. As a long jumper, he was unrivalled. But in the 100 metres, in my estimation, his supremacy was not certain. I now thought I could pose a real challenge to him in the not-so-distant future.

I won two bronze medals in the 1984 Games, one for the 100 metres and one for the 4 x 100 metre relay. I still have these medals today. They remain in the record books.

A few days after the Olympics, I had another opportunity to beat Carl Lewis at a European meet held in Zürich in August 1984. It was a race that I thought would work to my advantage because all the world-class sprinters were gathered there including Lewis, Calvin Smith and others. This kind of competitive field motivated me, spurring me on to improve even more. According to the rules of this tour, established celebrity sprinters did not have to compete in the preliminary heats. They would go straight to the finals. Not so accomplished runners like me, on the other hand, had to battle through the heats and through the semis, before getting to the big moment. The competition was very stiff. But I was up to it. I ran hard and earned a place in the finals. My muscles were tightening up again but I was not about to give in, not now.

Learning from my experiences in Los Angeles, I knew it was imperative to get off to a good start this time, avoiding any possibility of a false start. The plan worked and I was well ahead of the pack after the crack of the pistol. I surged even more down the middle of the track. I went out with such speed, I felt as if I were alone out there. "Where was everyone else?" I wondered. Curious, I glanced back to see. I was six metres from the finish. In a flash, Lewis flew by me followed by another sprinter, Harvey Glance. That's right! Glance! My glance had cost me the race. I clocked 10.12 that day, a new Canadian record and still I came in third. Lewis ran a time of 9.99 and inexperience had gotten the best of me once more. My poor judgment cost me the race. This was the sixth time I lost to Lewis.

To lose to Lewis was no disgrace. But to lose to Glance was something else. Glance was a respected competitor. He won gold as a member of the USA 4 x 100 metre relay team in the Montréal Games in 1976. But I thought he was a non-contender in a much younger field. This goes to show that experience cannot be discounted. Glance went on to repeat a gold medal victory as a member of the USA relay team at the 1987 World

Championships in Rome. His durability has to be respected, but so too his experience. Experienced sprinters do not look back. I did and it cost me the race.

I asked Bryan why I was so driven to win, or more to the point, why I had such fear of failure. He responded by telling me he had already discerned this issue, privately on his own. I was surprised. He said he was glad I was asking the question: The answer would allow me to better understand who I am. Bryan explained I had fear of failure because I had a very difficult time overcoming loss and I did not want to be known as a loser. He also said there was a part of me that always wanted to be remembered in history. He said this really is the core issue of why I had fear of failure. These were my beliefs he said. These core beliefs became the fuel to drive my physical engine.

I sat there, thinking. After I had a moment or two to process this Truth, I realized it made sense and I had to agree with him. Bryan reminded me that this Truth did not come from him. It came from God Who works through him. As I continued to ponder this, I had to ask another question. "Bryan, what is my soul's definition of a loser?" Bryan shut his eyes and went to God.

Ben, you ask the question, what beliefs are attached to your soul that define what is a loser? For I must answer the question by saying, in God's Eyes, in God's Truth, there is no such thing as one being a loser. For the human experience has been set up for all My Children to learn about love and learn about forgiveness. Through each step of the spiritual journey, there is at times joy, at times great disappointment. There are lessons that all My Children go through in order to achieve the goal of being one with Me. The ones who lose are the ones who have much to gain; and the ones who win, yes, they often get a big lesson, as it happens time after time that the winners forget about Me, and the losers eventually embrace Me. I have taken much blame and many of My Children ask Me, "Why?" For most of My Children who ask Me, "Why," have too much anger in their hearts, preventing them from receiving Me. For even the winners shall eventually lose, and they too will eventually come back to Me. For the weakness in one is the strength to come back to Me.

That makes so much sense. My experience shows this is definitely true.

At the elite level of competition, it was all about winning. At this point in my career, I was in the thick of it. While I had lost to Lewis, I was still ranked among the top three and I knew my moment was near. The previous few times we raced, I felt I had dominated him, at least for the first 60 metres, forcing him to play catch-up. I could see the possibility that one day he might not be able to catch me.

On May 11, 1985 I lost to Carl for the seventh time. It was in Modesto, California at the beginning of my outdoor season. Carl and other members of the American team had the good fortune of being able to train outdoors weeks before. This was not possible for the Canadian team, so we were at a great disadvantage. However, I was determined and I was not going to let this discourage me.

Carl ran a blistering 9.98, while I ran 10.16. But I still had confidence in my abilities. I knew my accomplishments earlier in the year were exceptional. I established a new Canadian record by running 6.56 in the 60 metres at the invitational meet in Osaka, Japan. This inspired me. I also did well in Paris in the inaugural World Indoor Games. Despite a hectic travel schedule and jet lag, I came in first, beating Sam Graddy. Later that same month, I competed again in New York at the Milrose Games, followed by yet another performance at The Toronto Star Indoor Games. These competitions gave me great exposure and experience but the traveling was considerable. By the time Carl and I met in May, I was pretty well exhausted. I was not in optimal condition. I had virtually flown around the world in less than a month and competed in more than eight competitive races.

Victory over Carl eventually came in Zürich in August 1985 during the European tour. Although my start was not spectacular, my endurance and speed work were now clearly paying off. I went with Calvin Smith head-to-head for the lead. I held my form and won the race in 10.18 facing a strong headwind. Smith finished second in 10.19 while Desai came in third. Where was Carl, I wondered? I did not look for him during the race but afterward I discovered he had finished fourth. I was not surprised I was able to beat him but admittedly I was surprised by his performance.

I wanted very much to compete with Carl again following my victory over him in Zürich. It was important to establish that my success against him was not a fluke. But our paths would only cross again once more in 1985. I ran in Berlin a few days after Zürich but he was not there. I did see him in Cologne shortly thereafter, where we both ran a mediocre race to come in second and third. I also ran at the World Cup in Canberra, Australia in October that year. Carl, also expected to show, was nowhere to be found. At the World Cup, I won in ten seconds flat while running into a headwind.

With all my achievements in 1985, however, Lewis was still regarded as the King of Speed. He had now become known as "King Carl." It was reported he had earned more money that year than in all previous years from his endorsements. He had a celebrity status, on and off the track, which was impossible to ignore. I was not surprised, therefore, when Track and Field News ranked him in 1985 at number one in the 100 metres and myself as number two. I was, however, disappointed. To be convincing, I realized I had to beat him again. In order to convince everyone my accomplishment was not simply a stroke of luck, I had to continue to be a force on the track.

I asked Bryan to discern how my soul felt being number two. God gave me the answer:

Ben, you ask Me the question, how does your soul feel when you lose? Ben, go back to your childhood in Jamaica. Do you remember the first time that you ever lost? For you played that game with the stones, trying to get the stone to the closest mark. And remember how you felt when you lost? You went away very angry but not giving up on strategizing how to win the game. And you would eventually go back and win the game. For this is how you are programmed: You believe you must win, Ben. But you never experienced any joy from the actual act of winning. Your joy was experienced knowing that you would not be called a loser. And if we were to go deeper, and venture together into your other incarnations, you would realize there is something you did in another life where you felt you could not be recognized as a winner. For this issue that is attached to your soul has to be healed. And once this has been healed, the fear of failure shall no longer be.

I chuckled and I said, "Yes, I need a healing."

The 1986 indoor season gave me the opportunity to begin to set the tone for the rest of the year. From that first race in Osaka, Japan in January, I did not look back. The 6.50 seconds I ran in the 60 metres was an improvement on the previous year and this time, I was able to establish a world record in that event. I won five or more such races straight, an indication my block work was in place and I was becoming more consistent.

The outdoor season opened in San Jose, California. It was May 31. When I arrived in San Jose for the Bruce Jenner Classic, I was shocked to discover there had been no reservation made for me at the hotel where all the athletes were arranged to stay. I was annoyed but I did not think much of the mix-up at the time. I was anxious and miserable after a long flight. I was tired and needed to rest before the race which was scheduled for 4:30 that afternoon. I promptly requested a hospitality suite but my request was denied because there were no meet officials available to confirm my reservation. The hotel refused to agree to my request. I sat, annoyed, in the hotel lobby until about 2:30 p.m. when other athletes and meet directors began to arrive. No one was ever able to provide me with an explanation as to why no reservations had been made on my behalf. After much ado, I finally was given a suite at approximately 3:00 p.m. I had no time to eat or rest before the race.

Media interest was very high at this meet. Whereas previously, the American media had largely ignored me, now I seemed to be on their radar more frequently. They portrayed me in negative terms, making me out to be a "Johnny-come-lately" who was jealous of Carl's accomplishments.

I asked Bryan about the media's portrayal of me, fearing he would confirm that I was jealous of Carl Lewis. Through my experiences with Bryan, I know it is impossible to lie to him. After discerning, Bryan confirmed that there was jealousy registered on my soul toward Carl Lewis. I asked him to explain where this jealousy came from. Why was I jealous of Carl Lewis? Why was I mostly jealous of him and not anyone else? The Lord explained:

Ben, you are asking Me the question, where did your jealousy come from, the jealousy that you have toward Carl Lewis? For what I am going to say next will, again, be a stretch for many. For this Truth I am about to reveal is for the purpose of your soul and Carl Lewis's soul being healed. For the healing must take place to stop the ongoing rivalry between both of your souls from one incarnation to the next.

For both of you go back to the core reference life, back in Ancient Egypt. For Ben, you were a great ruler and Carl Lewis was your son. As ruler you always wanted to be worshipped and acknowledged. It was your son who took this desire of being worshipped away from you. In that life, he took your life by poisoning you.

So today, the rivalry continues. For you believe Carl Lewis took your life in such a way it felt like you had died. For this memory is locked in the fractured soul that is attached to your soul. This memory is locked in the fractured soul that is attached to Carl Lewis's soul. For yes, there is much more to be revealed, but this is not the time.

I always wanted to go to Egypt and see the big pyramid. Now I understand a deeper reason for this attraction to Egypt I sometimes feel. Everything the Lord said made sense to me.

It was difficult for me to ignore the media and concentrate on what I was in San Jose to do. But I was determined to stay focused on what really mattered: winning my race. When the gun went off and the race began, I took the lead and never let it go. I won easily in 10.01. Rumour was Carl had been suffering from knee problems. With this victory, I finally started to be taken seriously and given respect by other athletes and officials. However, in order to erase any doubts, later that year I won against Carl Lewis again, twice.

The intensity and emotions were now high. Carl could no longer ignore me. His public comments now centered on "kicking ass," namely mine. Carl and I exchanged words that today I regret. Checking with Bryan, he said Carl did not have any real intent to harm me. He just got caught up in the hype, like I did.

I asked Bryan to ask God, "Is it registered on my soul that today I do regret what I said?"

Ben, you ask Me if your soul has regret for how you and Carl treated each other. For My child, for most of My Children do not understand what it means to have regret. For your spiritual journey has allowed you to come a long way. Today, you take self-accountability and self-responsibility whenever you bring harm against another, and you have regret.

But I will say to all My Children: not more than 5% of you take self-accountability and responsibility. Therefore, not more than 5% of the total human population is truly able to have regret when they bring harm against another. The future of the world, this planet called Earth, is dependent on all My Children developing the ability to have regret.

On July 9, 1986, I reached a significant personal milestone when I ran under 10 seconds with a time of 9.95 at the Goodwill Games in Moscow. My start was not even perfect. Lee McRae had that benefit. Still, I raced past him and all the others to win. Chidi Imoh of Nigeria came in second while Carl came in a distant third in 10.06 seconds. Carl did not attend the medal award ceremony which surprised me.

On reflection, it occurred to me: My hotel mishaps were coinciding with highly publicized races in which the media portrayed Carl and me as fierce competitors. My hotel experience in Moscow at the Goodwill Games was again less than desirable. Larry had confirmed my reservation ahead of time and I made sure to arrive in Moscow nine days before my event just in case there was any problem. But unfortunately, the assigned hotel left a lot to be desired. The food, the accommodation, the distance from and transportation to the track were all less than adequate. The food was unappetizing. The bus to the track was always late. Sometimes, the driver did not even show up. Impatiently, Charlie and I often would take a taxi to the stadium in order to have enough time to complete our training program.

Still, I made the best of it by blocking out all these distractions. I must admit I was not pleased when I learned Lewis's camp was staying at the American Embassy in Moscow. There, they could prepare for the competition and live in relative comfort. Despite the problems we experienced off-track, I won that race, setting a new low-altitude record.

On August 13 at the European Grand Prix held in Zürich, I repeated the victory. I was not expected to do well there. After the Goodwill Games in Moscow, I had competed in numerous meets including the 1986 Commonwealth Games in Edinburgh. There, I won two gold medals in the 100 and the 4 x 100 metres, and bronze in the 200. It was grueling. I competed again in a dual meet between Great Britain and Canada in early August and I placed fourth. A few days later, I ran a 200 metre race in which I came second. By August 13, I was completely exhausted, my body worn out.

The media hype persisted in Zürich and I now realized this was something I had to learn to tolerate. It was not going to stop. With my growing popularity, fans as well as journalists would often appear from nowhere. I felt like I could not move without someone approaching me to talk about one thing or another. I was not used to this and took it casually at first.

I remember while riding in a courtesy car in Zürich on the way to the track, there were others in the vehicle with me. One fellow who seemed very laid back began to casually interact with me in a way that appeared as if he were trying to befriend me. I had seen him around before but did not know who he was. He was keen on going clubbing later on, and asked me if I was interested in going with him, implying he knew a lot of women. I later saw him again while I was warming up and would see him frequently around the track. We did go out to a club together that night and it was obvious he was popular with the ladies. His name was André Jackson. Little did I know André had more in mind than just having fun. Today, even after everything that has happened, I completely forgive him.

I asked God, why is it important for me to forgive André?

Ben, you ask the question, why is it important for you to forgive André Jackson? For deep within your soul, you do have the answer. Ben, as you have learned through many sessions with Bryan, when one forgives another, the one who does the forgiving truly gets the greater benefit. For it takes one of courageous character to forgive another, and it takes a coward not to. The one who is courageous and forgives has no fear of moving on to new experiences, allowing one to spiritually grow to a higher level. The one who chooses not to forgive is fearful of moving forward and having new experiences for them to spiritually grow. For you and André Jackson and even Carl Lewis go back to the original life when you were Khufu, a pharaoh of Egypt. It is this life experience that has brought all three of you together and that has brought many others together.

Forgiveness is very difficult for most of My Children to go through because they have forgotten much. There was a time when the pineal gland was the size of a golf ball which allowed My Children to have greater recollection of other incarnations. Through the journey of My Children, they have become further away from Me and as they become further away from Me, the pineal gland has shrunk to the size of a pea.

It is important for you, Ben, to cut the cords of suffering. For those who refuse to forgive, refuse to forgive others, for most of them have a belief that they must suffer to be received by Me. Again, this is not the Will of God. For this is man taking on the role of God and making My Children believe falsely.

For I say to all My Children: How am I able to forgive you if you have not forgiven another? I say to My Children: Follow a path of resolution for oneself and for others. For if you follow a path of resolution, only for yourself, and not for others, for you will not be received by Me. And when I say follow a path of resolution, I mean follow a path that minimizes one's own suffering and minimizes the suffering of others.

Even My Children, who say that they pray, do not understand what it means to pray. For if you pray for good will for all, it is meaningless if there is no effort, sincere effort, to help others. For I say to My Children: prayer without sincere action is worthless.

Lined up to start the Zürich race with me were Carl Lewis, Chidi Imoh, Calvin Smith, Linford Christie, Kirk Baptiste, Harvey Glance and Marian Woronin. If I was worn out and tired upon my arrival in Zürich, I wasn't anymore. I summoned the energy to win. Imoh came in second, while Lewis finished third. This time I did not cramp up, nor did I look back. Instead, I closed in on the finish line and just kept running until I crossed it. I raised my arm in complete delight.

As a result of this win, the media went into a complete frenzy. The Lewis-Johnson battles were now like heavyweight matches. I had trumped Lewis convincingly more than once. It was my time: I knew I had proven myself on the track and had demonstrated it by performing much better than I ever had before. My race times were significantly better. I told myself I was just racing against the clock. I was not threatened by Carl.

I began to experience the circus-like nature of this business. I remember in Zürich how Carl arrived at the press conference in a limousine. I felt uncomfortable watching Carl arrive on the scene, looking very much like a rock star. He offered up all sorts of excuses for his loss, including the weather and a wide assortment of injuries. He also took the opportunity to speak about his singing and dancing career. He seemed poised to give up track and field for a new career in the entertainment industry.

Today, I realize I have a deep soul connection with Carl. We have had a long soul history together. I know that there are still outstanding issues between us that need to be healed. Bryan discerned that throughout my running career, Carl had empathy for me. On a soul level, he never wanted to hurt me. I certainly wish I had that clarity many years ago.

At the end of 1986, I was ranked number one in the world in the 100 metres by Track and Field News. It was an acknowledgement of my hard work. I believed I was well on the way to reaching my potential. The truth is it was my time.

I asked Bryan to discern if my attitude toward Carl Lewis in the 1980s was unfair. I asked him to ask God about this.

Ben, you ask Me if your attitude toward Carl Lewis is unfair. Ben, allow me to remind you, any weakness that you see in Carl Lewis, the same weakness lies within you. Instead of speaking poorly of Carl Lewis, use Carl Lewis as a barometer, as a measurement to know, to determine when your soul has been healed of those weaknesses that you see in Carl Lewis. The day you look at Carl Lewis only with love, that is the day you know your past, and you know your soul, have been healed.

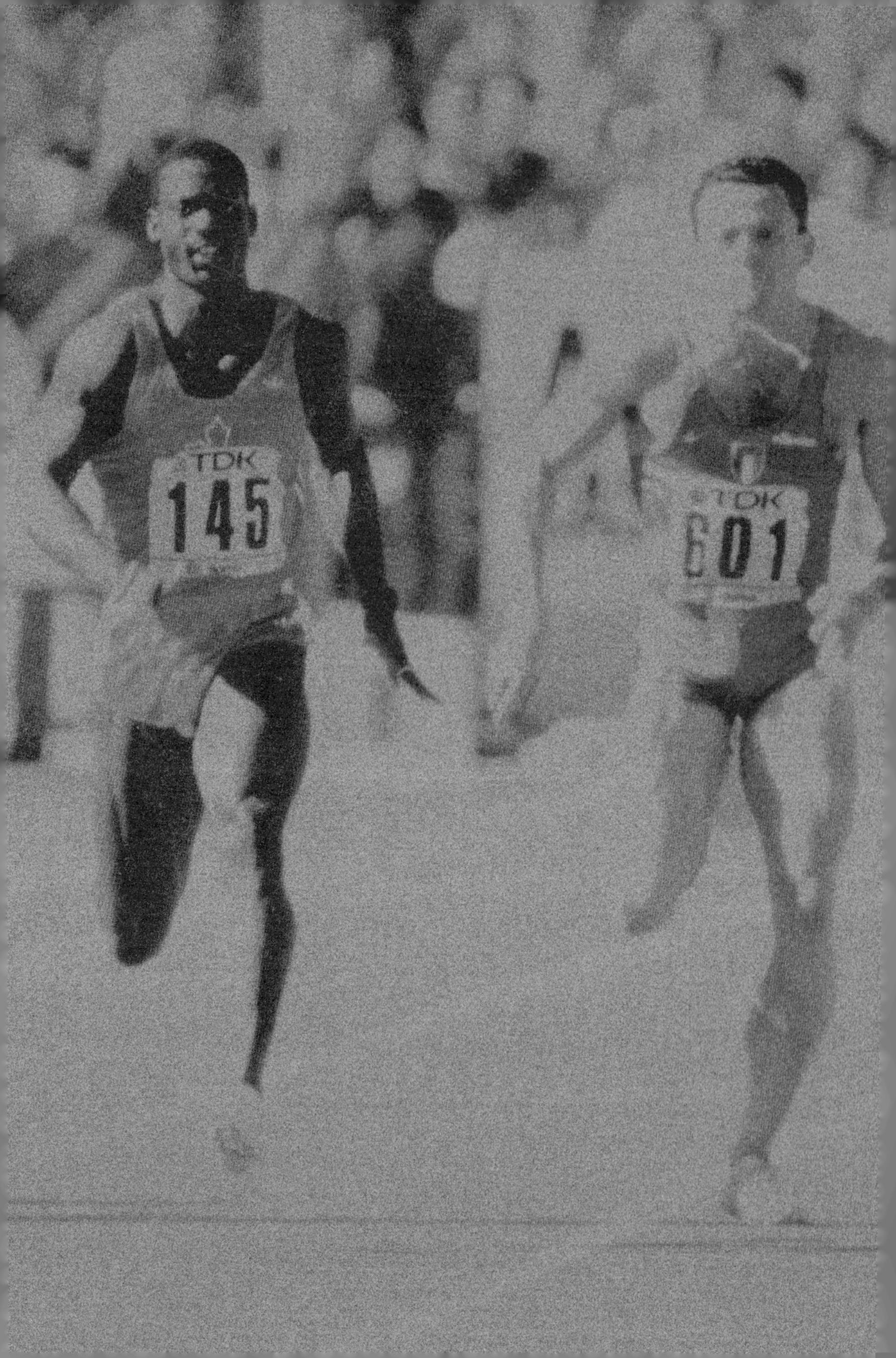
TDK
145
TDK
601

CHAPTER 10

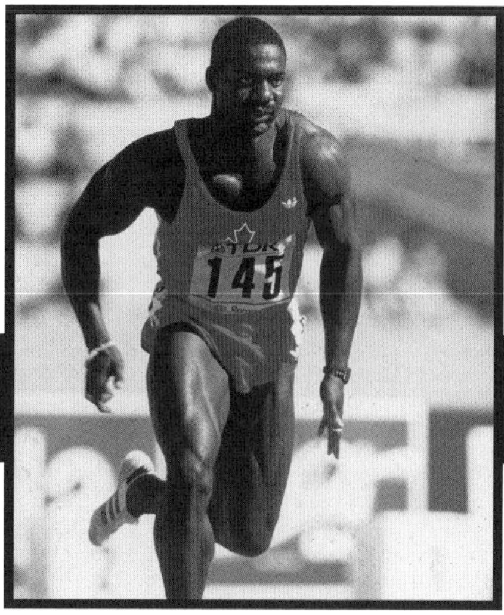

Rome

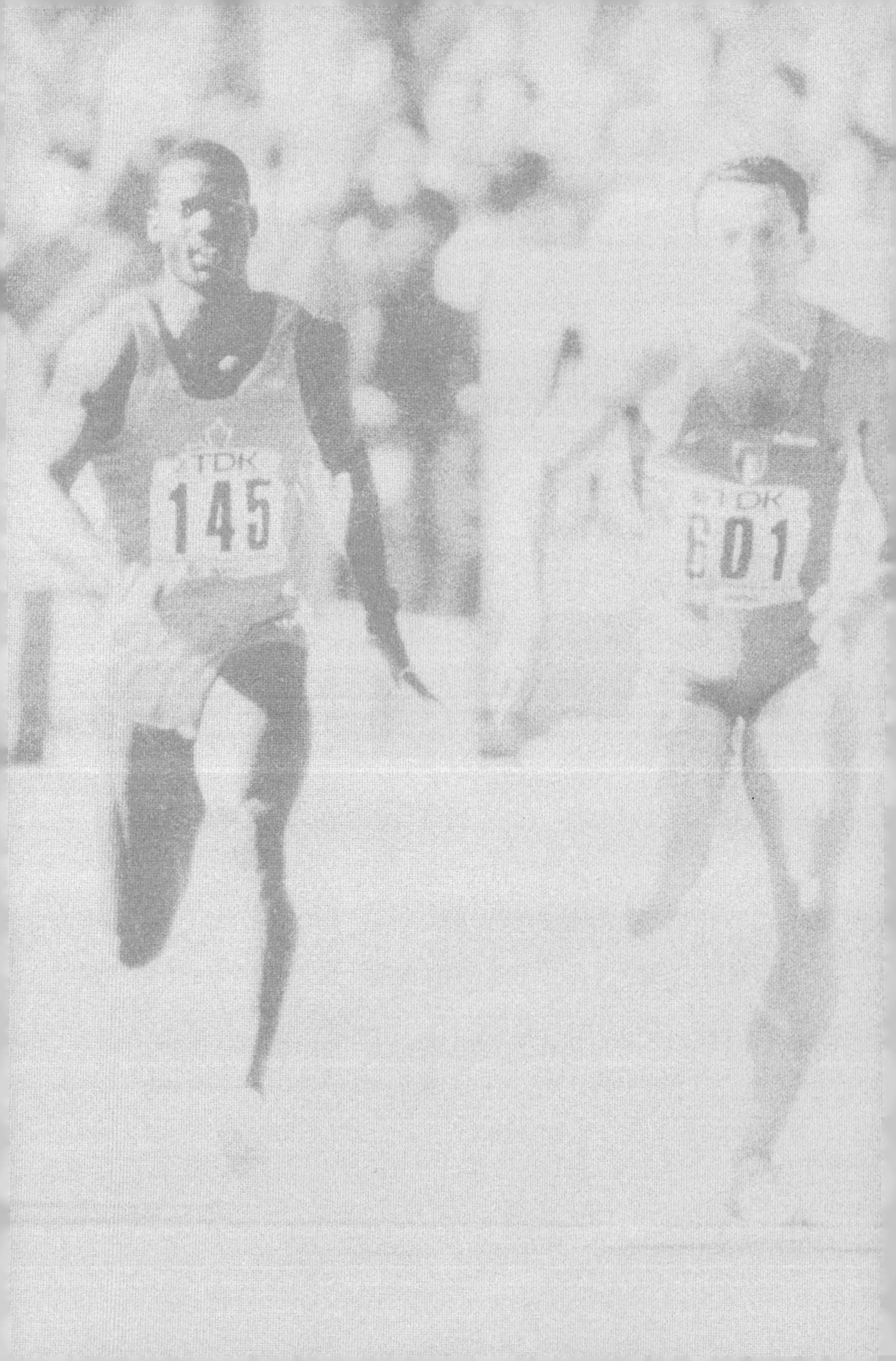
TDK
145
TDK
601

CHAPTER 10

Rome

Rome, Italy, August 30, 1987. Sunday afternoon at the World Championships. When I was younger, my mother made sure all six of her children went to church. Instead, here I was, on the mondo at Stadio Olimpico in Italy. What is my mother thinking right now? ... Bryan would later discern she was nervous, as always before a race. My start is so quick and she feared I would be called for a false start... She is watching me. She is in the stands with the other thousands watching, lost in the crowd. I cannot see her but I know she is there. I can feel her gaze as I prepare to run this race. It is as much hers as it is mine... Later, others would say my race was for them, too. But when the others withdrew from me, it was my mother who would stand by me... I know she is praying. I wanted to tell her to pray with her eyes open. For if she prays with her eyes closed she could miss me. But I forgot. I will look for her afterward.

It was hot, just the way I liked it. And there was a slight breeze. I sat in my blocks, carefully coiled, ready to go. There was excitement all around. I was calm. Sixty minutes before this moment, I was napping. Ten years before this moment, I was dreaming. The moment had arrived. I was ready, agitation all around. Everyone was nervous and jittery, except me.

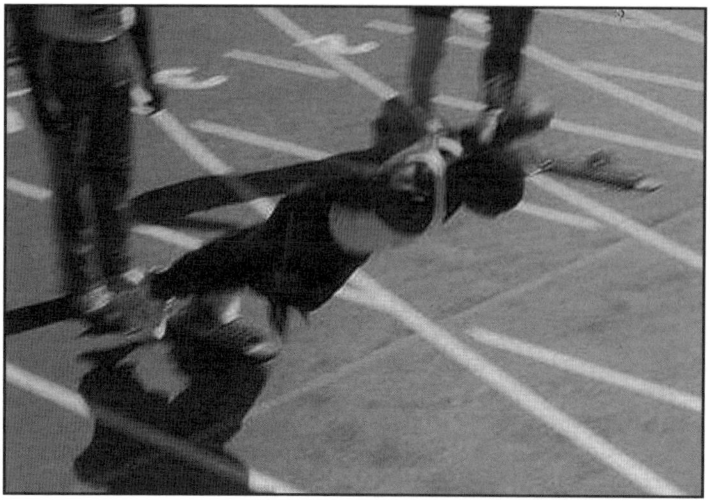

I felt like I was alone. But I wasn't. There were seven others who, like me, had earned their way to the finals. Fifty-one of us had started out. Now, there were only seven. There was the local Pierfrancesco Pavoni. Brave but injured, his quads were stiffly taped up. There was Viktor Bryzgin from the Soviet Union. He was known to be quick out of the blocks but he would not be the quickest today. I would. There was Attila Kovacs, the Hungarian national champion who had made a good showing in the semi- and quarterfinals.

Earlier, I was thinking how proud my mother and so many other Jamaicans must be. Ray Stewart was in lane three. He was a Jamaican who still ran for Jamaica. Linford Christie, also born in Jamaica, was running for Great Britain out of lane eight. And then there was me. I was proud to be born in Jamaica: I was proud to have the maple leaf on my chest and run for Canada. Today, I am still a proud Canadian.

And then there were the Americans, Lee McRae in lane seven and, of course, Carl Lewis in lane six. They had both beaten me before at various times. Today, I would win. Huge media hype surrounded this race. I was determined to win. But not because I was jealous of any runner.

Bryan confirmed, on that day I did not have jealousy towards Carl Lewis. Bryan went quiet and he closed his eyes. When he opened his eyes, he explained to me that even though the Lord comes through him on a continuous flow, after he receives the message, he confirms the information through the yea, yea; nay, nay process. And he said, "All the discernments I've done for you, Ben, have been done this way, as I always do with all my discernments. This is so that we all know, that we know, that we know."

Bryan continued and he started to discern the question I presented to him: What is the root cause of all jealousy? The Lord answered:

Ben, you ask the question, what is the root cause of jealousy? If one is completely with Me, one cannot experience jealousy. For jealousy is a source of much harm among My Children. Why would one have such jealousy? For one who is jealous of another is always jealous of themselves. They are looking at themselves in the mirror. They wish they were having the same experience, but feel unworthy to have it. For they had the same experience in another incarnation and thought they were not worthy and did not deserve it.

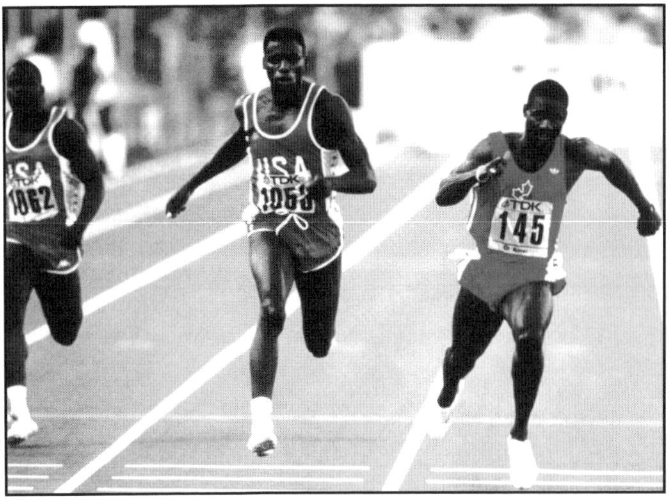

I was always motivated to win because I wanted to make people happy. I especially wanted my mother to be happy. I really wanted to make her proud of me because she had done so much for me. She always stood by me through thick and thin. Bryan confirmed this through his spiritual gift. He also discerned both Carl and I really did not want to be represented to the public as icons or be worshipped. I must admit, I truly believed that Carl did want to be the icon, at any cost. But Bryan discerned this was not the case. Like me, he only wanted to do his very best to win. Bryan said, "Both of you simply got caught up in the times."

Before I received this Truth, I had a different opinion of Carl, one that only brewed anger inside me. Hearing this discernment changed my perspective. The negativity I used to have simply dissipated. Compassion, and even love, began to replace my judgments. At times like this, I especially cherish my relationship with Bryan because his discernments help me to become closer to God, as God works through him.

Just before the race in Rome, my mind was completely clear. I wasn't thinking of anything. I shut out all the hype. I did not even hear the crowds or the other runners. The voice of the starter was all I heard. The silence was peaceful, the moment serene.

I was in lane five, right beside Carl. But I did not see him, did not even think of him, until close to the finish line when I popped him a glance. I had settled in, waiting, ready to spring, the sound of the starter's pistol my cue to drive. When the others got up, I was already gone, on my way to making history... 1987 was a good year... and 1988 was too.

All is vain: That is what my mother would say. And yet, it was hard to think I was not the fastest man on Earth. The honours and accolades kept on coming. Those who know me will tell you I don't often speak of my achievements. They speak for themselves. But it was hard not to become intoxicated with my success.

Some had called me a school drop out, made fun of my accent and stuttering speech and underestimated me. The actor James Earl Jones stuttered, as well as Ron Harper, a player with the Chicago Bulls. Rubin "Hurricane" Carter, who used his fists to discourage others from laughing at his stuttering speech when he was younger, also went on to accomplish great things. The limitations of speech did not stop them. And it would not stop me.

Here I was at age 26, a multi-millionaire just for being me, for being Ben Johnson. The hard work, discipline, sacrifice and commitment had paid off. But all seemed to be in vain. For when all was said and done, none of the awards and honours mattered. In the end, most would remember me not for my achievements as much as they would remember me for my downfall. But today, I know more than ever, all is not in vain. I am growing stronger.

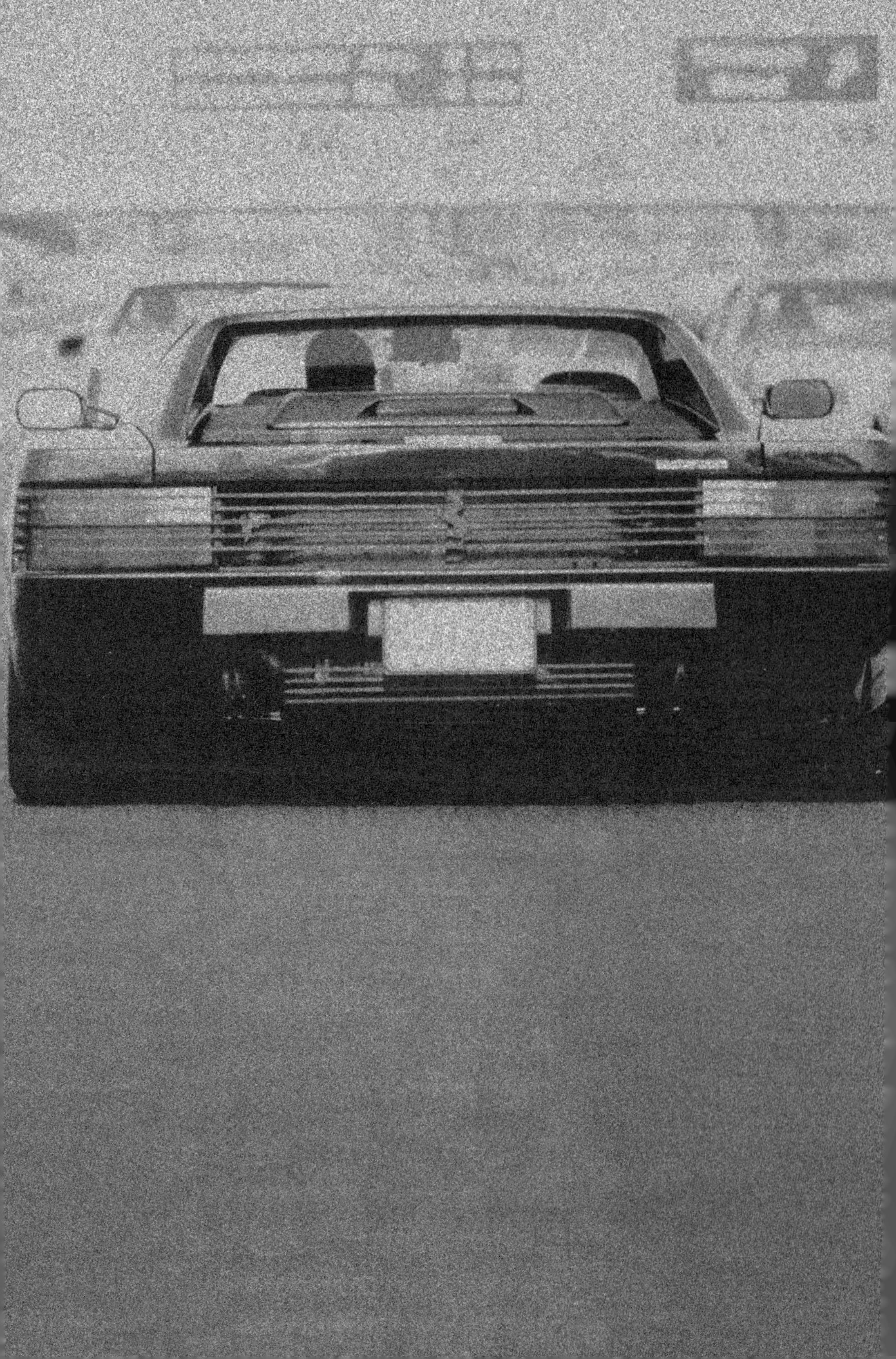

CHAPTER 11

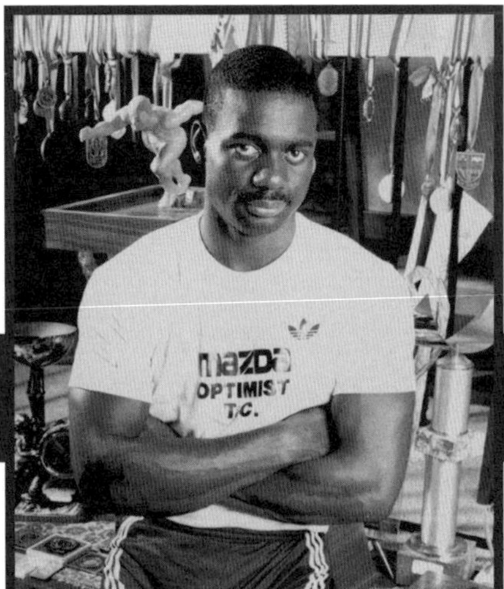

Being the Fastest Man on Earth

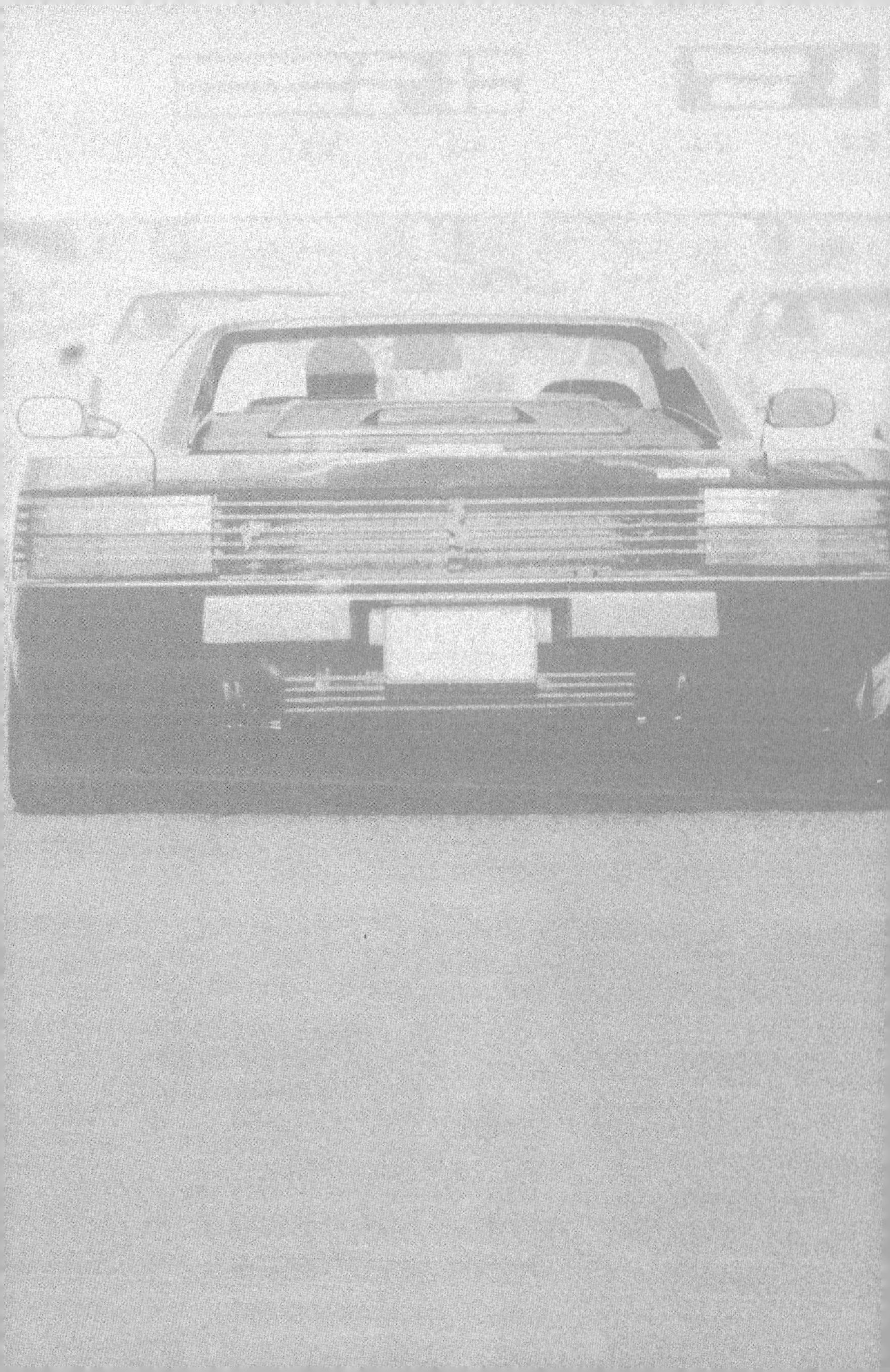

CHAPTER 11

Being The Fastest Man on Earth

"The higher monkey climb, the more him expose" is a Jamaican expression. It is a warning to those who succeed that they should be careful. Success brings new responsibilities. It can also bring new problems. This saying applied to me shortly after the World Championships in Rome. I had been doing well making a living from my athletic efforts. But after that one win, my world changed with a speed that would have been hard to imagine. It took me by complete surprise. Being on top of the heap was not as good as it looked because I immediately became a target.

The first sign of trouble came when Carl Lewis approached me after the race. The officials were still posting the race times when he ran over to grab my hand as if to shake it. I was suspicious because this was highly unusual behaviour for him. I was reluctant to return his handshake. My suspicion turned out to be right. Pretending to congratulate me, he looked me in the face and accused me of a false start. Later, the media made his act of shaking my hand seem like an act of sportsmanship. They did not realize his apparent gesture of goodwill was in fact an act of accusation. As I look back now, I realize this one act was very revealing. I did not have a great deal of experience with the media, but there were others who did. Not only is elite sports about achievement, it is about media hype and public perception. And Carl knew this.

Three days later, again through the media, Carl cast aspersions on my victory by suggesting it was performance-enhanced. I felt I was in a no-win situation. My

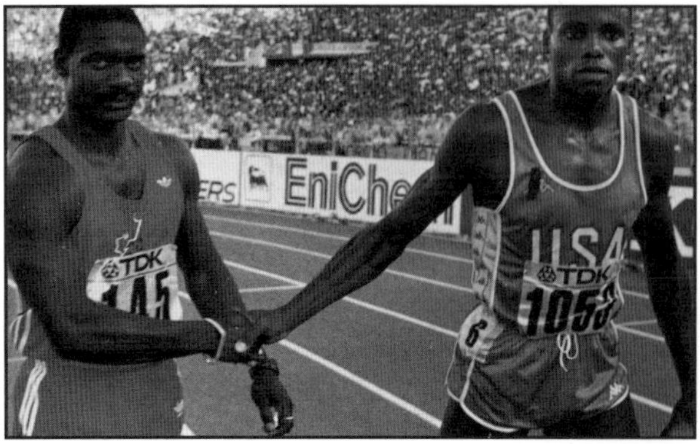

stuttering got in the way of me being able to express myself, so I routinely stayed away from the media. I did not feel comfortable dealing with these false accusations against me through the media. So, I ignored the attack on my character and stayed poised. I just wanted my family and our team to enjoy and celebrate the victory. Little did I know, many people were going to misinterpret this as guilt on my part.

Beating the world record quickly introduced me to new challenges in life. When I was declared the fastest man on Earth after competing in Rome, I was ill-prepared for the pressure and invasion of privacy that would come with having such a title. Not only was I now the fastest, but some predicted I would also become one of the richest. The days following my victory were the most hectic I had ever experienced up until that time. Everybody wanted to be a part of who I had become. From teammates, handlers, and fans, to media and sponsors, everyone wanted a piece of me.

In 1987, I was given many prestigious awards, including Male Athlete of the Year, the Jesse Owens International Award, Performance of the Year Award, and Top International Sports Personality of the Year. Canada also applauded and congratulated me by appointing me to the Order of Ontario and, much to my surprise, to the Order of Canada. I felt honoured to be appreciated in this way by my adopted country. I was proud to represent Canada. But it soon became clear to me there would be a price to pay for the recognition I had been working so hard to receive.

Everyone now expected to benefit from my new fame. So many people stood by me to get to this point. They, too, deserved to be rewarded. Some people were resentful, while others were envious. My new fame made it easy to attract new friends but it also made it easy to make enemies. I realized very quickly I had gone from simply being a sprinter to becoming an employer. People had to be paid. Some wanted a raise. Some merely wanted recognition. Still others felt overworked. This experience proved to be a very overwhelming time for me because I am not a personnel manager. This is not a skill God gave me. I had to rely on others to manage the people around me. So, I put my trust in certain individuals to make sure people were treated fairly.

My life suddenly went from doing what I loved and was passionate about to being big business. That transition was very stressful. Many sports figures and athletes go through this. Some handle it better than others. But it is not easy for anyone.

In the early eighties, sponsors began to acknowledge the attraction of track and field role models and their ability to promote products and services. With this appreciation, meet organizers began to substantially compensate athletes financially in the form of appearance fees. This was becoming more common when I made my arrival on the track circuit.

The CTFA, now Athletics Canada, created the Athletic Reserve Fund (ARF). This was intended to be a trust fund, administered and managed by them on behalf of athletes who were required to deposit their earnings into the fund. Earnings received from meets, sponsorships and interviews were now required to be deposited here. Under the governing sports body's rules, it was mandatory for all Canadian amateur athletes to deposit any and all earnings derived from their sport into the fund, until such time as the athlete either retired from the sport or died. This ostensibly enabled the athlete to maintain amateur status and eligibility to compete at IAAF-sanctioned events. If an athlete were caught breaching these rules, such as not depositing endorsement money or appearance fees, he or she could jeopardize his or her amateur status and subsequently be disqualified from future competition. The intent was to assist young athletes who did not have the experience in managing their financial affairs and this sounded like a good idea at the time. However, I later found out that my own ARF was mismanaged, not unlike how the NHL players' pension fund was reportedly mishandled. Once I became a world record holder, this brought in a tremendous amount of sponsorship money to the fund.

This challenging year was a time of transition, overcoming obstacles and learning many life lessons. My new level of success separated me from the rest of my crew. I would not have been able to make it without them and I valued their contributions. But now I had many more obligations, aside from track and field, to think about including business meetings, contract negotiations, business trips and appearances. Before, training had been everything. Now, it was only a small part of a much bigger picture. I had a lot of juggling to do. I can understand how this new level of activity caused my group some anxiety. I, too, was experiencing anxiety and it showed.

As more was demanded of me, I also demanded more of those around me. I wanted them to adjust their schedule to fit into mine. When they refused, I became disappointed. I looked to them to affirm my success by giving me the time and attention I thought I deserved. The success had rushed to my head and made my expectations unreasonable. When they refused to accommodate my wishes, I felt let down. I did not want to be responsible for paying their salaries as simply employees. I expected them to understand my needs and help me to address them. After all, my success was somewhat theirs, too.

As for my teammates, it was hard to pretend that we were on the same level anymore. The interviews, media circus and financial interest completely separated us, as did the fact that I had achieved a great goal. It is easy to be supportive of teammates when you are all striving, but once someone reaches a level much higher than the rest, it becomes very difficult.

Today, I realize this way of thinking was not appropriate. I have come a long way and grown spiritually. Now I know compassion is the answer. Compassion is seeing things from another's point of view, loving your neighbour as yourself.

Of the many life lessons I learned that year, the bottom line was this: It is easier to have no expectations at all. Having no expectations means you cannot be disappointed, you do not get angry and you minimize the creation of bad karma.

I asked Bryan to discern, "How would God answer the question, what is karma?"

Ben, so you ask Me, what is karma? For many of My Children ask the question, what is karma? Karma is not "Eye for an eye." I am not a God that punishes. Instead, karma is a learning experience of understanding what you may have caused another to go through. It is a learning experience to gain wisdom on how your decisions may have impacted another.

For many world leaders, for many politicians, for many civil servants commit many to war. But if they had complete Truth, in all cases they would not commit so many to war. They would not support war. But these same individuals who commit so many to war, they believe they are making the right decision. Even on the limited information, the absence of Truth, they believe they are making the right decision. Again, they do not understand the full impact of war... the pain that a mother goes through, knowing she has lost her son... the pain that loved ones go through, knowing someone dear to them has been killed or wounded. For even when they come back with no apparent wounds, for they are wounded. For many have lost their souls. For many suffer dearly. For many went against their will. For these same individuals who have committed those to war, through God's Math Equation they will experience the same thing. For I have designed the process of purification of the soul, where the actual experience of learning the impact of one's decisions is necessary.

I have sent Bryan to help the world leaders to know Truth. For many have made war their own personal war.

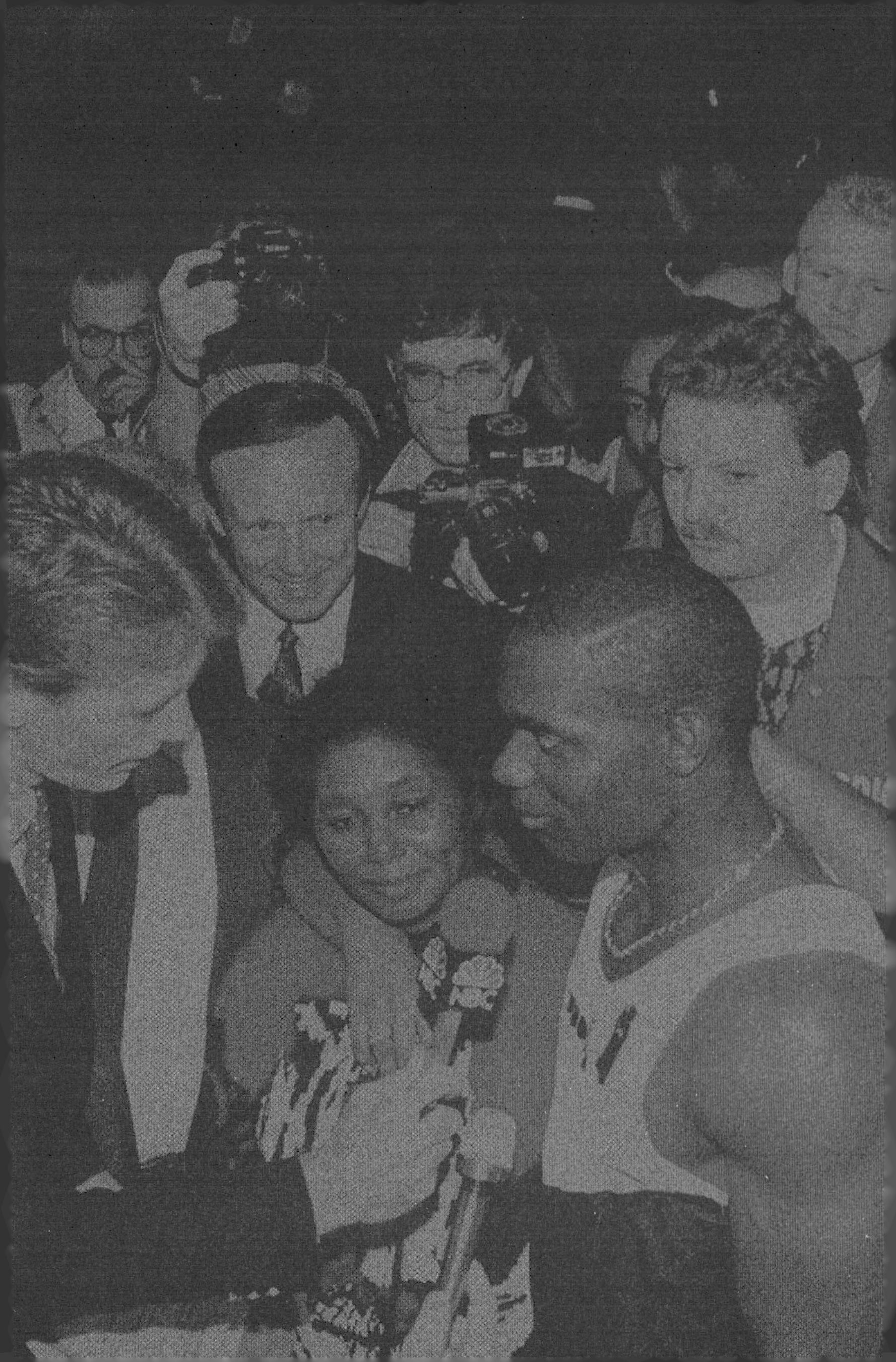

CHAPTER 12

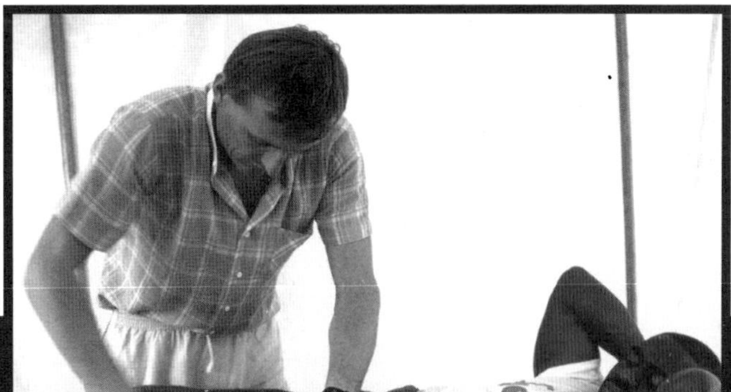

Fame and Injury

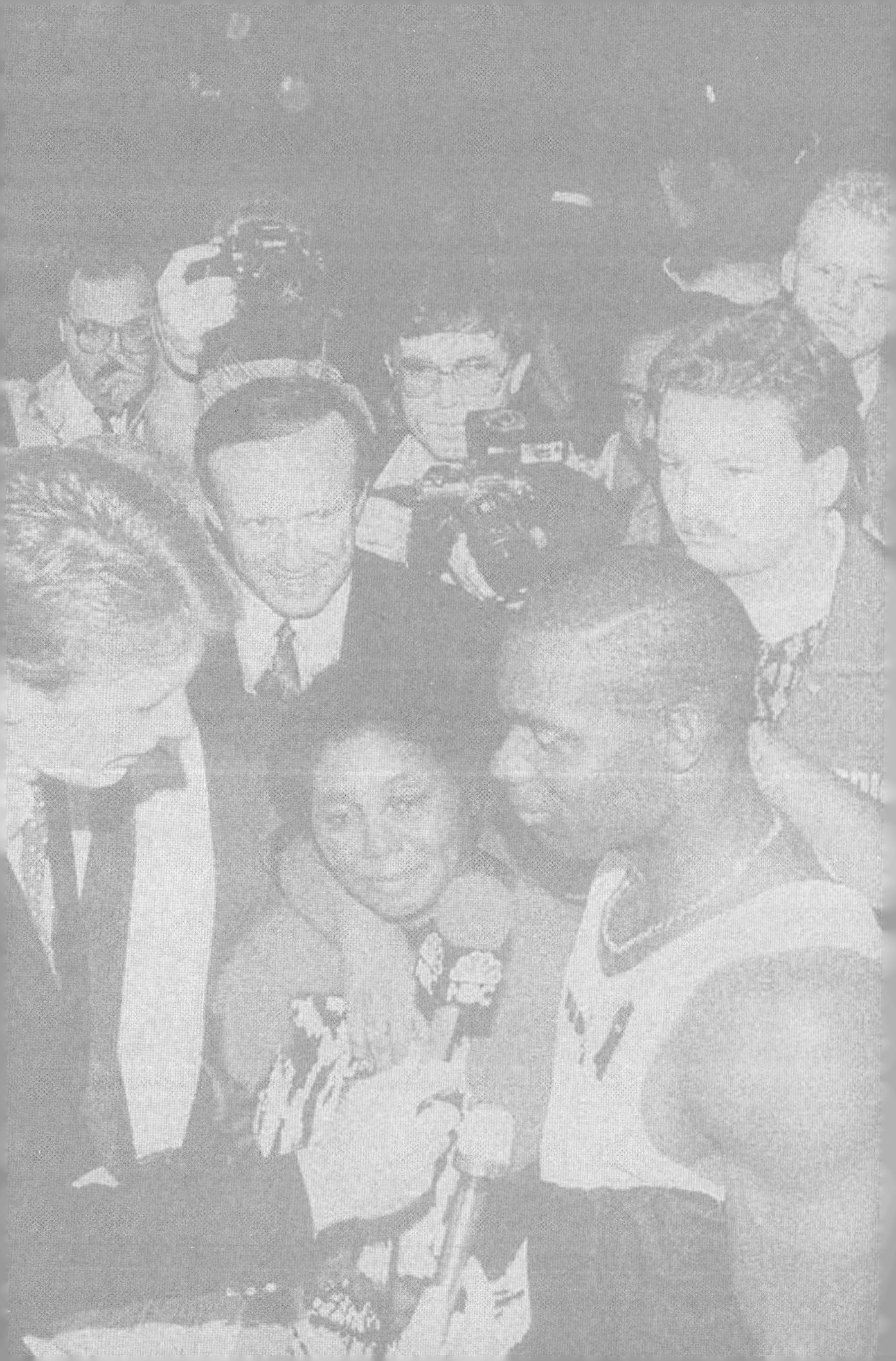

CHAPTER 12

Fame and Injury

When I boarded the plane to come to Canada in 1976, I had never traveled outside of Jamaica before. I had been to Montego Bay and even Kingston, the capital city of Jamaica. I had been in and around Falmouth where I lived, but otherwise, I knew very little beyond the shores of the Island. I had certainly never been on a plane. By 1988, in contrast, I had been to Brisbane, Caracas and Cologne; to Edinburgh, Helsinki and London; to Los Angeles, Madrid and Moscow; and to Prague, Rome, Vienna and Zürich, all because of my talent for running. The old man's prediction had come true. I was only 12 then. I was 26 now and I had come a long way very fast.

Many social opportunities came with my success. I met Prince Albert of Monaco, Her Majesty Queen Elizabeth II, Enzo Ferrari, Prime Ministers and Presidents, beauty queens and other celebrities. I asked Bryan how I really felt on a soul level at these times, as he can read me so well. He can read anyone so well. With God's permission, he can know us better than we know ourselves.

Bryan's calm response was, "Ben, you know at the most prestigious events you attended, you, at times, experienced nervousness. This was due to your fear of being rejected by others. This is why you worked so hard as a track runner: Because you did not want to fail, only to be rejected by others. And so, eventually, you were led to Seoul one day, for you to experience the fear you always lived with: You were rejected by so many. For this, Ben, was the ultimate blow to you."

And I have to agree, this is true. The good news? I asked Bryan, "Where do I stand today with my fear of failure?"

He responded, "For you no longer have fear of failure because you have overcome the lesson. You have learned: One is not to be afraid of embracing success and one must be prepared to embrace the disappointments that come with success. You, Ben, had fear of becoming very successful. You believed the more success you would achieve, the disappointments would be bigger: You believed you would be giving up something you loved for something else. The fear you had is that you would give up your mother and your family for success, for entry into the illusion of the material world. Part of you did not want the illusion of the material world if it meant you had to give up those whom you love."

In 1982 when I could afford it, I got my first car, enabling me to soar both on and off the track. It was a white Pontiac Trans Am with a big eagle emblazoned on the hood. Over time as my income improved, I raced through several different cars: two Corvettes, a Ferrari, a Toyota Supra, a Mazda 626 which I gave to my mother, and a Porsche 928. I do not consider myself materialistic: When it comes to cars, I do appreciate quality.

I had always wanted to own a Ferrari. In June 1987, I went looking for one at a local Toronto dealership. The manager at the time told me the waiting list for a Ferrari Testarossa was over five hundred customers long. My chance of getting one any time soon was not promising. But I was determined and would not take no for an answer. I told the manager I would be back very soon to pick up my new car. I had a feeling I would have a Ferrari one day. And I did.

After celebrating my victory in Rome, I asked my agent Larry Heidebrecht to set up a meeting with Enzo Ferrari. Larry was always very resourceful and I had no doubt he would make this happen. While relaxing at the hotel after a hectic series of media interviews, I was thrilled to receive a call from Larry telling me he had a personal invitation from Enzo Ferrari. The date was set. Enzo and I met at his factory north of Milan where he told me, through an interpreter, how my speed at the race amazed him. He congratulated me on my performance. I in turn wasted no time in expressing interest in his cars. I told him of my visit to the dealership in Toronto and my dismay when I learned how long I would have to wait to own and enjoy one of his cars.

On hearing this, Enzo smiled and gave me a punch line he must have rehearsed several times in preparation for our meeting: He said in English, "The fastest man on Earth should have the fastest car on Earth." With that, I picked out a black metallic Testarossa with a black interior. Enzo said there were only three others ever built like it and mine would be the first ever black edition. He assured me the car would be ordered the next day with delivery to Canada scheduled within the year. He also advised me to return to the dealership in Toronto where paperwork would be waiting for me.

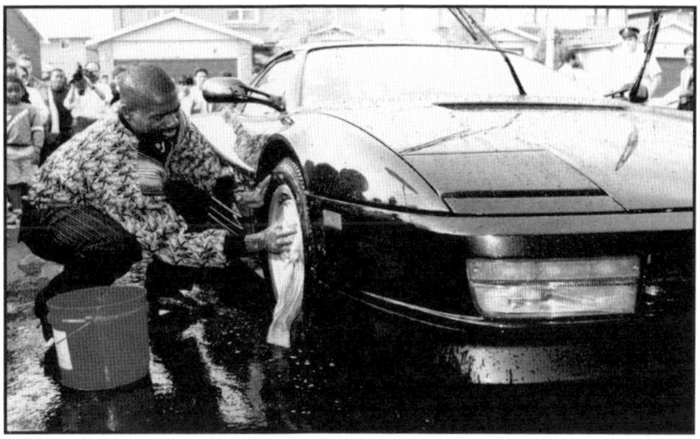

Sure enough, when I returned to Canada, all the relevant order forms were ready and waiting for me. The look on the manager's face when I walked into the dealership that day was unforgettable. He came up to me, gave me a quick congratulatory handshake for setting a world record in Rome, and wasted no time in satisfying his curiosity. "How the hell did you pull this off?" he asked. According to the manager, Enzo was known to decline special requests from royalty, celebrities and even members of his own family to make and build a car like the one I ordered. What I had done, said the manager, was exceptional. With that, we completed the paperwork much to my delight, the manager still in a state of shock.

I was so excited when my Ferrari finally arrived in the summer of 1988. When I got it, I felt like a kid. I knew everything about that car inside and out. Now that I am on a spiritual path, I have wondered from time to time why I was so attached to a car. One day, I got the idea to ask Bryan to discern how my soul felt about owning the Ferrari.

I was so surprised when he said, "On the day you got that car, you were happy. But, you were not happy because you had the Ferrari: You were happy because Enzo Ferrari had kept his word, his promise, and he delivered. The only other time you were happy with that sports car was the day you got rid of it."

Bryan went on to say, "Why would this be true? You did not feel comfortable driving anyone in that car. Even alone, you were not comfortable. You had fear of going too fast and getting into a serious car accident. More importantly, the car did not symbolize truly who you are. The illusion of the material world did not bring joy to your heart. The only person who really gave you joy was your mother and no one else. It was very easy for you to give up your Ferrari. But since the day your mother died of cancer, to lose that joy, it has never been easy for you."

This is true. My experience with Bryan has been truly amazing.

A personal invitation to my family and me came from Prince Albert of Monaco when I was in Monte Carlo at the Hôtel de Paris. The invitation came quite unexpectedly, hand delivered to me at the hotel. I gladly accepted this offer. The Prince personally picked me up in his Porsche convertible and invited me to attend a luxury car show in the Principality. We shared an interest in cars. I have fond memories of our meeting that day and consider myself fortunate to have had the opportunity to meet and spend time with Prince Albert and his family.

Three years my senior, the Prince was gracious to my family and me. He, too, would become an Olympian as a member of his country's bobsled team in 1988. He had been a member of the International Olympic Committee since 1985. Like Enzo Ferrari, he spared nothing in showing me European hospitality. The Prince received us with open arms.

If the Prince and Royal Family felt in any way that I let them down after the Seoul Olympics, I ask them to forgive me. I wish the circumstances were different. But it was not written to be, as Bryan advised me.

I asked Bryan to discern why God had me meet the Prince of Monaco.

Ben, you ask Me the question, why did you meet Prince Albert? For you and the Prince have had many other lives together. In some of the other lives, you did grow up together. For in this life, he is to help you, and that time is yet to come.

While in Rome, I also received an invitation from Pope John Paul II. However, for some reason the invitation did not come to my attention until it was too late, somehow getting lost in my new and overwhelming schedule of interviews, appointments and meetings. Why did his invitation, in particular, get lost? The question stayed with me. Having often wondered about the significance of this apparent miscommunication, I asked Bryan to discern the reason why I did not meet the Pope.

Bryan said, "It was the Will of God for you not to meet the Pope this time. It is the Will of God for no man to worship another man and for no man, like yourself, to expect to be worshipped. For the true God, the true Temple is only found in one's heart." He went on to say, "Those who accept this Truth will be blessed."

I asked Bryan to discern an even deeper reason why I did not meet with the Pope. God answered:

Ben, for you are seeking an answer to a question that requires one to have great wisdom and understanding to know the Truth I am about to give you: Since the creation of man, man has gone on his own path, and I have allowed this path to continue, although the path becomes much more difficult, as My Children have accepted a belief, a set of beliefs, that have fortified their relationship with man and not with Me.

For I have sent many Messengers throughout time to dismantle, to weaken these beliefs. Today, many speak of Me. They believe they speak of Me but it is not Me who speaks through them. For one cannot be truly connected to Me if one is not able to know Truth. Many Messengers I have sent through time have been denounced.

For now I send another Messenger and you know this Messenger as Bryan. For the path that you shall both go on shall be together in times and separated in other times. But both paths lead back to Me.

The task at hand is difficult. Religion teaches My Children division, that I am a punishing God. Through religion, My Children believe they are unworthy, that they are not worthy of Me. Through religion, My Children would rather be in a room full of people who experience misery than to be in a room of people who experience joy. For I am a loving God, a joyful God and I would like to see all My Children come together as one. For My Children should not accept that they are better than the other. They should not identify themselves based on the religious institution or any institution that they are a member of. They should simply identify themselves as a child of God.

I asked Bryan, "Is this not going to make people angry, hearing this Truth? Could you please ask God for the appropriate response to subdue one's anger?"

Ben, yes, it is true, that many will be very upset with hearing this Truth. Many will criticize. Many will judge. Many questions will be raised and even when the answers have been given, the Truth, they will still not accept. They will not accept because their hearts are full of revenge that they are consciously not aware of. For those who truly are of Me will know that these words are of Truth, are of Me.

Perhaps one of my most memorable meetings was with Her Majesty the Queen. I was amazed to meet her after I competed in the Commonwealth Games in Edinburgh,

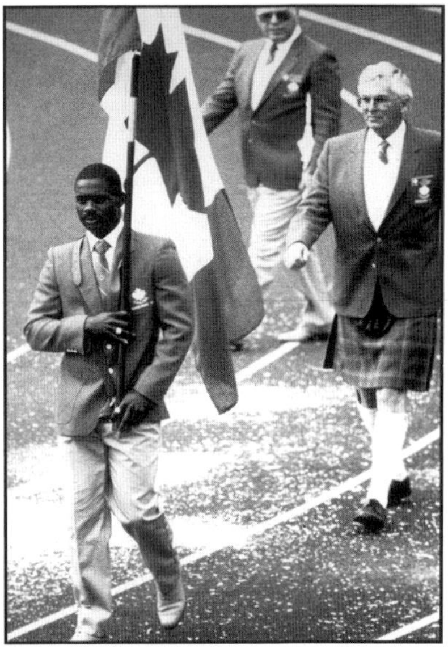

Scotland in August 1986. She presented me with the gold medal for my winning performance at the Games. The controversy that followed took me by surprise. The media had characterized me as being disrespectful because I did not bow when I was introduced. But I remember being humbled by the experience of meeting the Queen and feeling very honoured. I shook her hand with the biggest smile and a gleam in my eyes, a sign of respect and affection I usually reserved only for someone like my mother. I gave her a big heartfelt thank you.

The truth is, I was not informed or advised of the proper etiquette on how to address Her Majesty the Queen. The Queen nevertheless was very gracious and did not display any displeasure or disappointment with my breach of this special protocol. I remain honoured to have received the gold medal from her. If I did offend her, I ask her now to please forgive me if she believed there was any undertone from me suggesting that I did not respect her. I ask the people of Great Britain to forgive me as well.

I asked Bryan to discern why I did not bow down to the Queen when I met her. He replied, "Ben, all humans come into this human life experience, one of many, with master contracts that, on some level, control our beliefs and our total experiences. You came into this life... most human beings who have had other incarnations come into this life... with a fractured soul. The fractured soul has memory of one's past life including memory of one's false beliefs. You have gone through spiritual trauma, as many others have, in another incarnation.

"One will come into a new life with a fractured soul of revenge towards another if one has not forgiven all. And with this fractured soul, they will meet those individuals in a subsequent life to implement their revenge against another. At the moment of the revenge, it is the fractured soul that controls their response.

"So the process of spiritual healing requires all fractured souls to be purified through the act of forgiveness. And once the fractured soul has been purified, this fractured soul merges with your soul to become whole again. The one life God gives us is the total soul journey, all the life experiences we undergo from the original soul. If one truly accepts past lives, they accept full self-accountability and responsibility for their past actions.

"If one truly accepts past lives they will not express arrogance, skepticism, revenge and war. They will not hold on to false beliefs.

"So, what does all of this mean, Ben? You came into this life with a fractured soul, having anger towards the Queen. This fractured soul has been healed and you no longer have anger towards the Queen. You have forgiven the Queen. You have forgiven her soul completely.

"You came into this life, as many others have, with a master contract not to idolize anyone and to worship only God. This master contract is important for you to have so that you did not have your spiritual path compromised by giving your power over to another. Whenever someone has power over another, in every case, they have revenge toward another. Remember, the most powerful can often be the most revengeful."

I looked at Bryan and God began to speak:

Ben, the spiritual journey to Me cannot be compromised by hanging on to religious false beliefs. For the journey to Me is a very difficult path. For true redemption is not found in the spirit realm. True redemption can only be accomplished through the experiences of the physical realm... again, not in the spirit realm. One cannot be truly redeemed if one holds on to false beliefs. One cannot be truly redeemed if one wishes to have power over another. One cannot be redeemed if one has revenge toward another.

I asked Bryan to ask God, "What does it mean to be redeemed? I don't understand."

Ben, for you ask the question, what does it mean to be redeemed? It means when your soul is completely cleared of all false beliefs, of all that separates you from Me, that prevents your soul from completely being purified... when you are free of all of this, this is what it means to be redeemed... to eventually become one with God, joy to joy with God.

As I looked at Bryan, he responded with a humorous smile, "For many people do not understand why the Dalai Lama has so much laughter. For they will say the Dalai Lama is not of God. This man is of God."

Following the 1987 World Championships in Rome, I went into overdrive. Despite a hectic schedule, I closed out the season in perfect form winning all of my races, 21 straight victories. In the month of September alone, I ran and competed in seven games. The 1988 winter indoor season opened with a similar pace, with similar success. In February, I accompanied the team on a European tour which included Spain and Germany.

In Sindelfingen, Germany, while I was midway through and accelerating in the semifinal of a 60 metre run, I injured my hamstring. I won the race but lost the ability to run again for the remainder of the indoor season. It was my first serious injury since I started track and field in 1977.

I asked Bryan why I got the hamstring injury in Sindelfingen. God answered:

Ben, you ask the question about your hamstring injury. For you came into this life with a false belief that if you did not show appreciation to Me, to God, that you must punish yourself. It is not My Will for My Children to punish themselves if they do not take time to appreciate Me. The appreciation that I look for in My Children is expressed when they love one another as I love them, as I love all. This is the true feeling of appreciation.

I was without words.

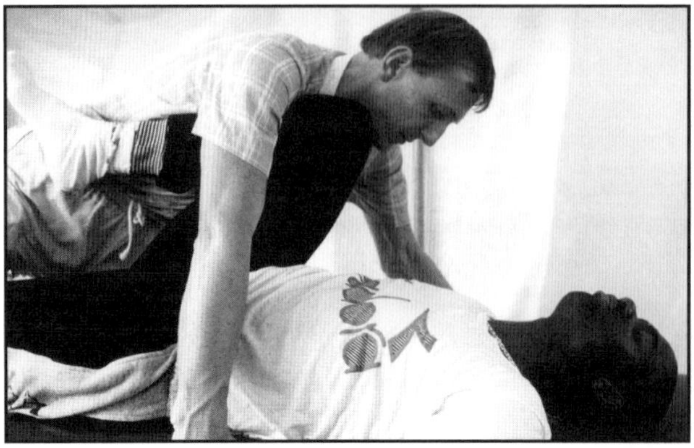

I stayed with the team for the rest of the European tour, getting therapy and treatment from Waldemar. The promoters of the tour still wanted me present to capitalize on my popularity and build attendance. They knew I would be a draw for the crowd. I was not able to run and the promoters understood. Unfortunately, two days into the tour, I was injured again, this time off the track.

While I was visiting a city called Karlsruhe in the southwest of Germany for a media photo shoot, a group of German children swarmed me for autographs. I was knocked to the ground during the scuffle and I got kicked in the leg, the same leg I had injured.

This kind of attention followed me to Genoa, the last stop on our European tour. Although I had become more cautious, dodging the chaos when I could, I was still hounded by hundreds of people who would come looking for me. It became so crazy, it was necessary to arrange a police escort. I was not able to walk around anywhere alone. I was easily recognized and my mother prayed for my safety.

By the time I returned to Toronto, I was exhausted. I just wanted to rest and relax. I needed some time to myself. My leg was only 80% functional. But I had to train because the outdoor season was just around the corner.

The first outdoor race was in Japan. I was told about requests from sponsors in Tokyo that I needed to strongly consider. Over the past few months, I had traveled to Japan frequently for business. These trips interrupted not only my training but also my physical therapy treatments. Nonetheless, this trip was very important for business reasons and could not easily be ignored.

In Japan, my popularity had grown way beyond my expectation. I had major endorsement contracts there. The Japanese business people paid me upfront for most of my appearances. Taking the money and not showing up was not an option for me and would have been irresponsible. My mother, who often gave me counsel, would have disowned me if I did not follow through on my commitment. So, I took the 48-hour round trip flight to Japan, like I had so many times before. Except this time, I was not in very good shape. My hamstring was still in recovery and I still had trouble lifting my leg. From an athletic standpoint, it was not a good decision. From a business perspective, it was necessary.

Making the trip to Tokyo and my decision to compete there was disastrous. At the meet, I got up when the gun went off, but got up much slower than I normally would. I did not want to apply too much force to my injured leg. Even though I was running, I could not shake off my opponents. Instinctively, I then decided to go for it and run a little faster. Shortly after accelerating, I felt excruciating pain. I stopped and limped off the track. When I was rushed to a hospital in Tokyo, the doctor who examined me said part of the muscle had torn away from the bone. This was very serious and could have ended my career.

Running with this type of injury was, of course, impossible. Meet organizers who were expecting me to run at their event were understandably worried because they depended on my participation. Finding somebody to replace me was not going to be easy. To ease their worry and prevent the organizers from losing money, Charlie and I agreed we would not say anything publicly about the extent of my injury. We decided to only say the injury was being treated and evaluated day by day.

Just when I thought things could not get any worse, they did. Sport Canada, a branch of the Federal government, put out a news release saying I was injured and I would be out for some time. The public reaction was one of surprise. Promoters and organizers began calling us, demanding an explanation and full report on my condition.

They felt we had deceived them, double-crossed them. They did not understand we had nothing to do with Sport Canada's news release. They were upset the news went public before they were informed directly.

The situation became very tense. I was told I would not be able to recover fully from my injury until the beginning of summer at the earliest. The Olympic Games were scheduled for September. Our preparation time was slipping away fast. Charlie had one idea about how we were going to proceed. I had another. He wanted me to go with the team to Europe where Waldemar could work on my leg during the course of the tour. However, Charlie's insistence that I go to Europe at this time did not sit well with me. I also did not like Charlie's attitude toward my injury. I did not think he understood how I was feeling about it: I was scared.

For a split-second, I had the thought: This injury could end my career and my dream, ending all I worked so hard for. I was determined for this not to come true. At the time, I felt as though Charlie and some other members of my team treated the situation as a risk worth taking to keep bringing in the money. I do not think they understood the pressure I felt and the toll it was taking on me. I was disappointed when I noticed certain members of my athletic management team did not show enough compassion for what I was going through while I was healing my leg injury.

I later asked Bryan about this situation. He said, "Ben, despite any negative rumours through the media about Charlie Francis, I have discerned that Charlie Francis really loved you. He tried his best to protect you and making money did not drive him. It was his love of the sport and the love he felt for all the athletes he helped that drove him. You must never look at this man poorly."

I agree. Bryan further discerned that Charlie Francis was born with a master contract to treat all his sprinters equally. However, at the time, I thought Charlie still regarded me as a scrawny boy in high-tops, simply just one of his sprinters. But back then, I felt the stress and pressure of trying to live up to an image: the fastest man in the world... a celebrity. I did not think he realized this. How could he? I had not quite come to terms with it myself. He did not completely understand the stress I was facing, not to mention the fatigue associated with 11 years of intense training and traveling.

Consequently, Charlie and I could not agree. After 11 years, this was the first real disagreement between Charlie and me. Instead of going to Europe with him and the team, I stayed back in Toronto and enjoyed some quality time with my mother. She suggested I take a vacation. So, I packed my bags and went to St. Kitts, at the invitation of Dr. Jamie Astaphan and his family.

I have learned through my experiences with Bryan that there are no accidents. Even injuries have a spiritual significance. So, I was curious about the deeper reason why I got this injury. I asked him to discern it.

"Ben," he explained, "you had to go through this injury because it gave you time alone. Your soul needed this time so you could realize God's Hand was guiding you. During this time, you realized you had not been giving God the recognition that God deserved. Even as your muscles began to heal, there was a change in their structure that allowed you, on your own, without the use of performance-enhancing drugs, to run faster. For even the scientists who are caught in their realm of theory will not understand this statement.

"So, always look at this moment as a gift and realize all those around you at that time had their own master contracts that caused them to interact with you according to what is written in their master contracts. Embrace all. Forgive all. And love all. Do not judge, for we simply judge ourselves when we judge others."

I have forgiven all.

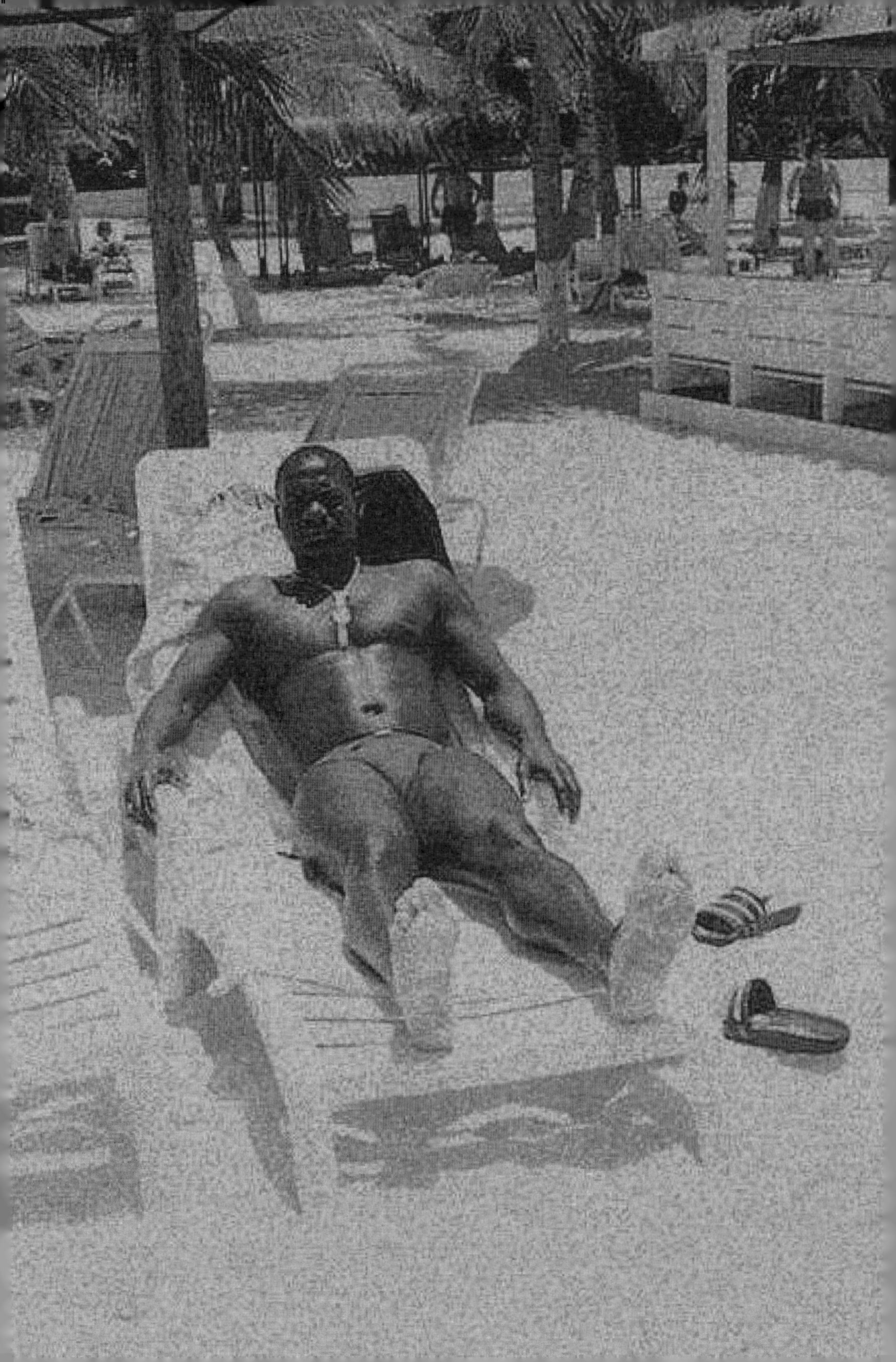

CHAPTER 13

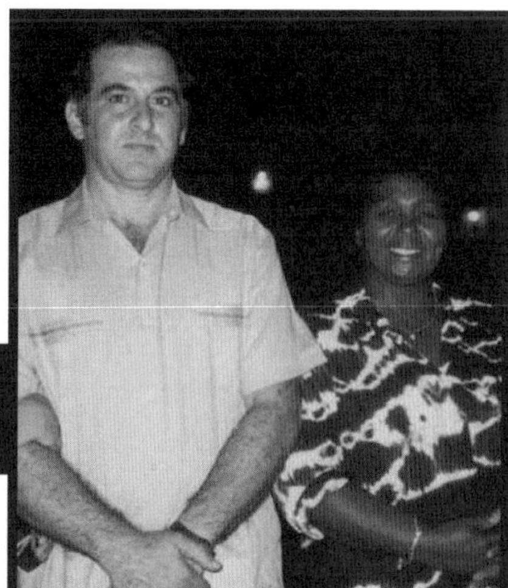

The Calm Before the Storm

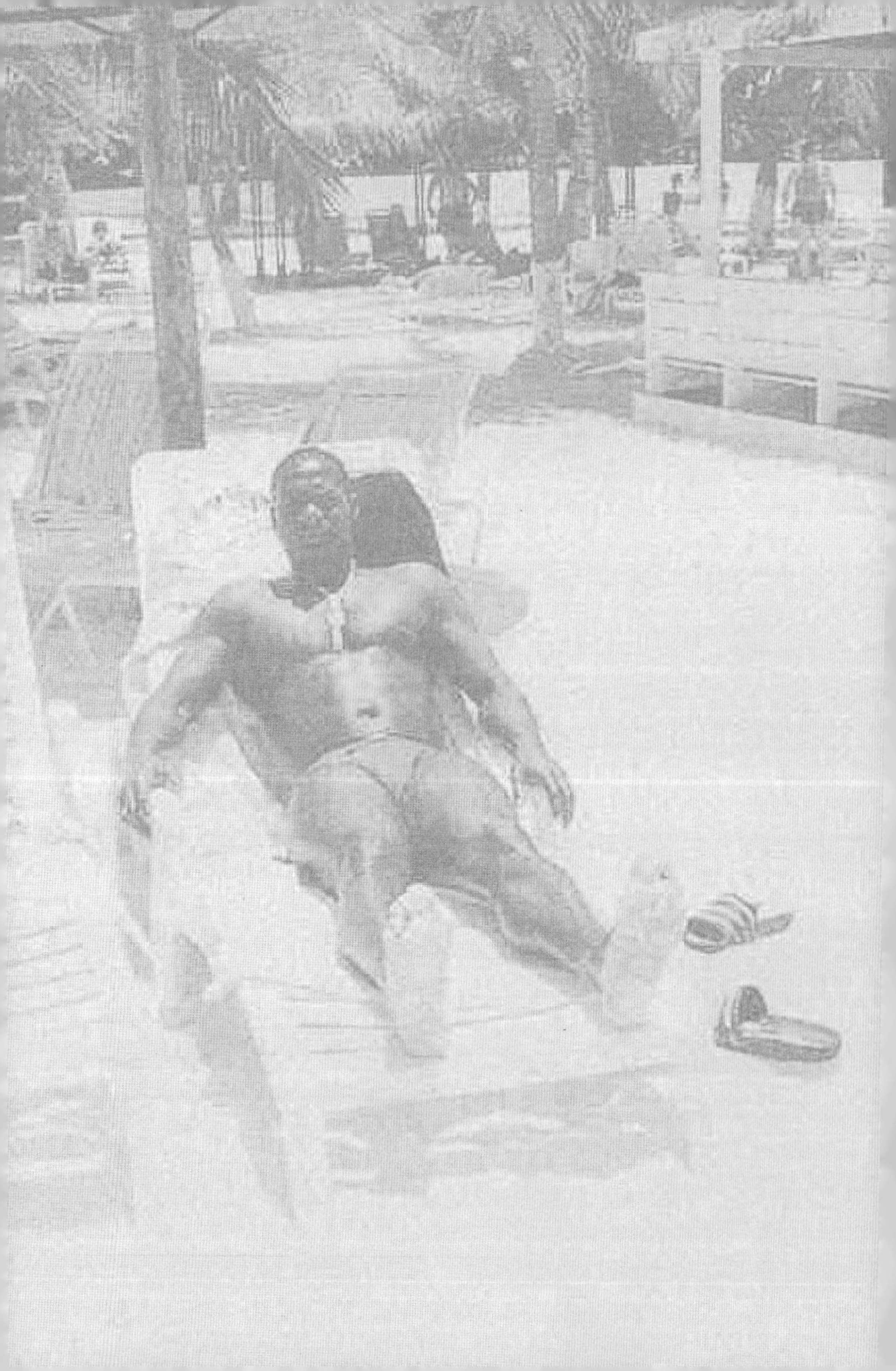

CHAPTER 13

The Calm Before the Storm

From the first time I met Jamie, I found him to be good-natured. I would visit his office sometimes two times per week for my injections while I was training. Originally from St. Kitts, Jamie was professionally trained in Toronto. It was Jamie's and Charlie's job to make sure I was properly monitored.

I never paid Jamie throughout the time he treated me. I do not know if he received money directly from the Optimist Club for his services or not. He liked to joke, "If you don't take it, you won't make it." Jamie always felt that if he did not personally provide me with steroid injections in a safe professional environment, I would be exposed to more harm elsewhere. As far as he was concerned, he considered himself to have been doing the right thing. Over time, we developed a friendship. I was particularly close to Jamie's younger brother, Kris. Jamie moved back to St. Kitts from Toronto in 1986. When he invited me to visit in June 1988, it was hard to resist.

Contrary to popular belief, I did not visit St. Kitts with the intent of receiving steroid injections. I did, however, receive treatment for my injury. This treatment included pills and injections prescribed by Jamie. I never really queried as to what they were. Because my trip to St. Kitts was later criticized by many, I asked Bryan about this. I asked him to discern what was really going on. What was the Truth?

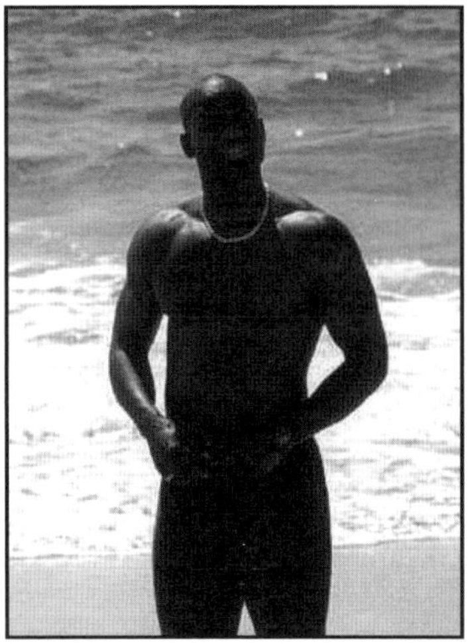

Bryan said, "Ben, as you recall, you had an injury that needed much rest and recovery. I have discerned that you did have a master contract to go to St. Kitts and receive steroid injections to help your recovery. For the world must always remember: Steroids will help one recover faster from injury and training, but steroids do not help one run faster. And you know, Ben, in the media, you will still be accused of being able to run faster because you have been able to recover faster. But the Truth is, steroids, in your case, only help you recover for not more than one day. On the second day, the steroids have no benefit for you, Ben. This would mean, to get any claimed benefit from steroids, you would have to take steroids a day before any race. But in reality, if you took steroids the day before a race, the muscle tightening effects caused by the steroid would actually cause you to run slower, not faster."

I asked Bryan to discern the situation surrounding Dr. Jamie Astaphan and Charlie Francis giving me the steroid injections. "Ben, I have discerned that God gave you a master contract where you did not need steroids to be the fastest man on Earth. It was difficult for you to say no to Jamie and Charlie with respect to taking steroid injections. When you were born, you were given another master contract that you trust others 100% until the time they have demonstrated that you can no longer trust them. I am not saying Jamie and Charlie are bad people. They had their own master contracts to fulfill. Their master contracts required you to go through the experience of steroids. Charlie and Jamie simply played a valuable role for you to spiritually grow. One might ask: How does this experience of taking steroids allow me to spiritually grow? The spiritual lesson, Ben, for you to learn, is that strength comes from one's inner self, not from one's outer self, meaning the inner self that God gave you was much stronger than steroids could ever make you."

So, I looked at Bryan and asked, "Why are so many in the media upset with me due to the fact I did take steroids?" Bryan discerned and then God answered:

Ben, you ask the question about steroids... why are some in the media upset with you? Ben, remember My son, what have I been telling you? Stop for a moment and pretend that you are a mirror. Now, imagine for a moment the members of the media who are upset with you. When they look into the mirror Ben, who do they see? Are they seeing you, Ben? Or are they seeing themselves? For the Truth is Ben, those who call you a cheater have looked into your mirror and they only see themselves. For their soul has memory of themselves being a cheater. For when they look at you, they have passed judgment on you with limited information, only to conclude with such limited information that you are a cheater. For you remind them of the anger that they have towards themselves of being a cheater. For yes, it is a misperception: Those in the media who call you a cheater, their anger is not at you. It is at themselves. For all of these individuals who call you a cheater must go on a spiritual journey and heal their own souls. The day when they can look at all and not accuse anyone of being a cheater, this is a sign that the issue that was on their soul has been healed.

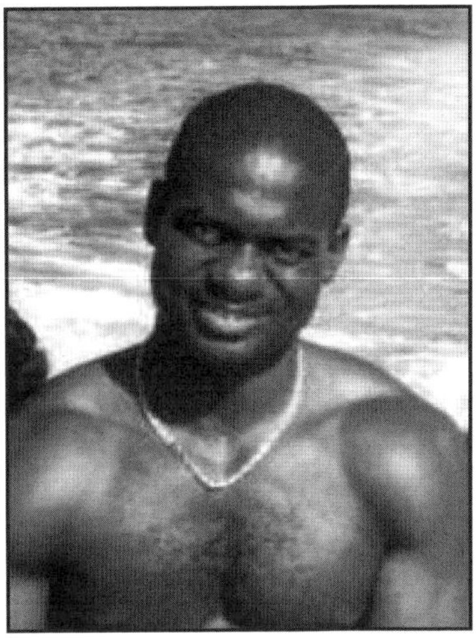

Ben, remember... always remember: Steroids do not cause one to run faster. They did not make you run faster.

Jamie's treatment plan also included water resistance exercises which allowed me to get in the water of the beautiful Caribbean Sea once again. Doctor's therapy or not, I had the most wonderful time, spending seven glorious weeks there. It was great not to have to worry about training and the intensity of being on the track circuit. Instead, I relaxed, had fun and allowed nature to rejuvenate me. I went to the beach every day, soaking up the heat and the salt water. I was like a little boy again. It was a great vacation. It would have been hard to see or imagine that in a few weeks some of the worst days of my life were about to unfold.

The weeks in St. Kitts revitalized me. When I left the Island during the second week of July 1988, I was in near perfect shape. Little did I know it was the calm before the storm.

Upon my return to Toronto, the tension between Charlie and me built to a head, not immediately but over time. For a while, neither of us said anything, avoiding each other as much as possible. It was awkward, two men trying not to lose face, but each wanting to renew a relationship. And then one day we went head-to-head. Charlie was upset with me and poured it on. He criticized me for not staying with the team, for not wearing my Diadora tracksuit, as my contract required, and on, and on. He was talking to me like I was a spoiled child. Then I, in turn, criticized him for not checking in on me while I was recovering in St. Kitts, for Waldemar's failure to prevent my second injury in Tokyo, for not listening to me, for making me feel guilty for wanting some time off, and on, and on. I found myself talking to him like I was a spoiled child who had missed his father, wanting his approval. I was disappointed he had not called to see how I was doing the entire time I was gone. He knew I was injured and under a lot of pressure. But still he did not call, not even once. It saddened me at the time. I thought he did not care.

I asked Bryan about my father-figure relationship with Charlie. Bryan discerned that I did look up to Charlie as a father figure, as my biological father was not there for me. This is a common phenomenon that athletes have with their coaches: Over time a strong bond develops. In my case, Bryan told me that a very strong bond developed between Charlie and me. I know this is true. My life experience fits perfectly with Bryan's discernment. I know he speaks the Truth.

Charlie and I had a long history together as coach and athlete. But our relationship grew to be more than that. Many times I would go over to his house, just to hang out. I would raid his fridge or engage him in small talk about cars or music. Other times, we would actually talk about track, training regiments, races I should run, races I shouldn't, and events coming up on the circuit. For as long as I could remember, we had communicated almost every single day. We had been together for the past 11 years or so. With the Olympics rapidly approaching, we both knew what had to be done. It took us only a few days to realize that our partnership was not over. At the end of July, Carl Lewis won a race in Paris in a time of 9.99, declaring he was running "better than ever" and that I was not running at all. Charlie and I knew it was time to pick up where we had left off. It was not hard to make up after that.

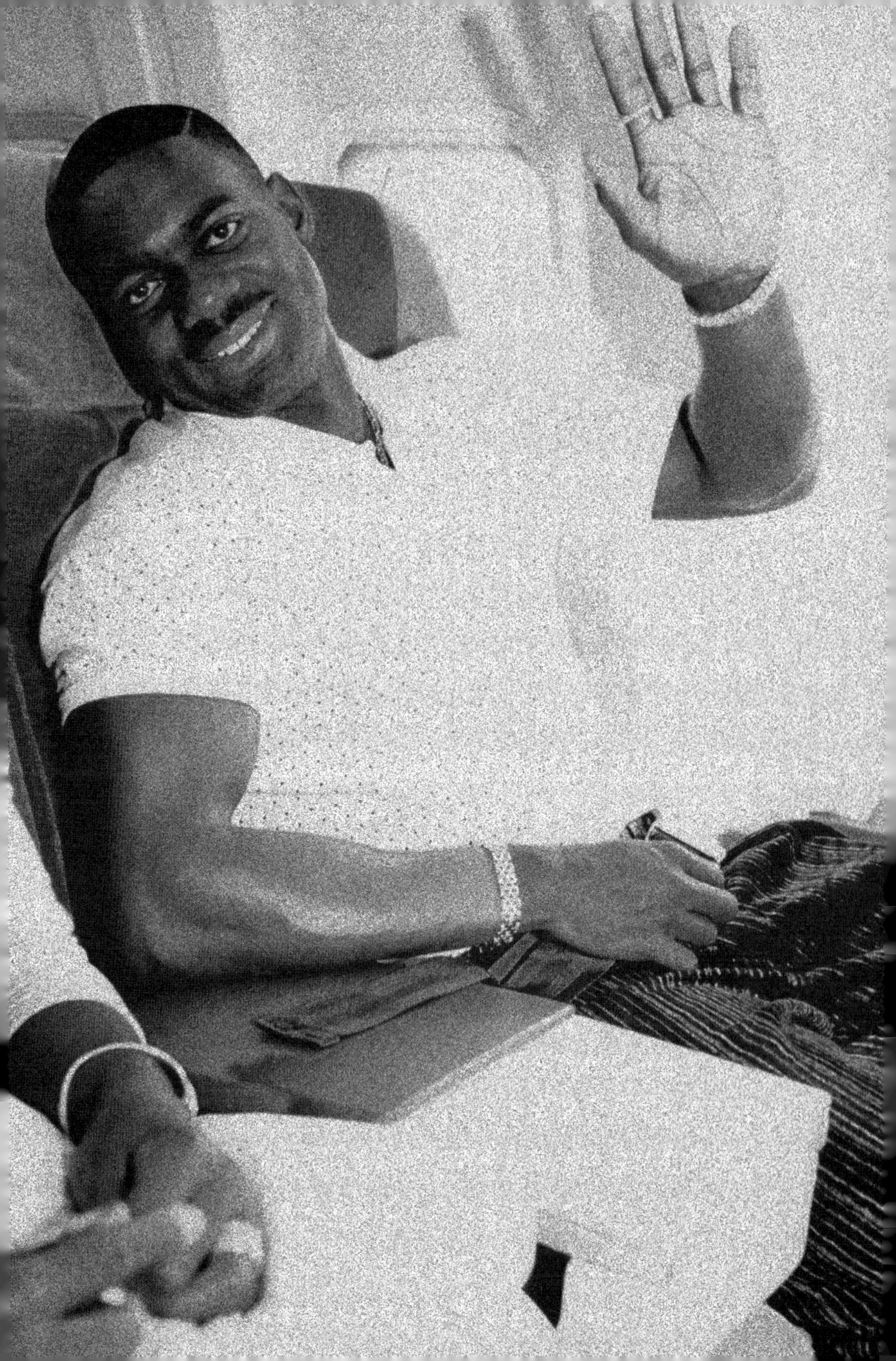

CHAPTER 14

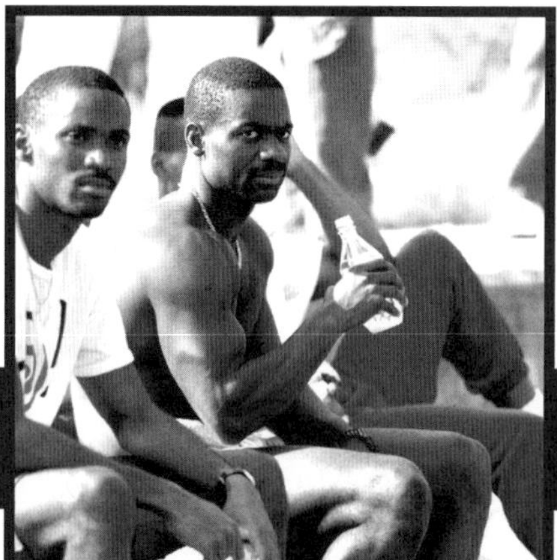

On To Seoul

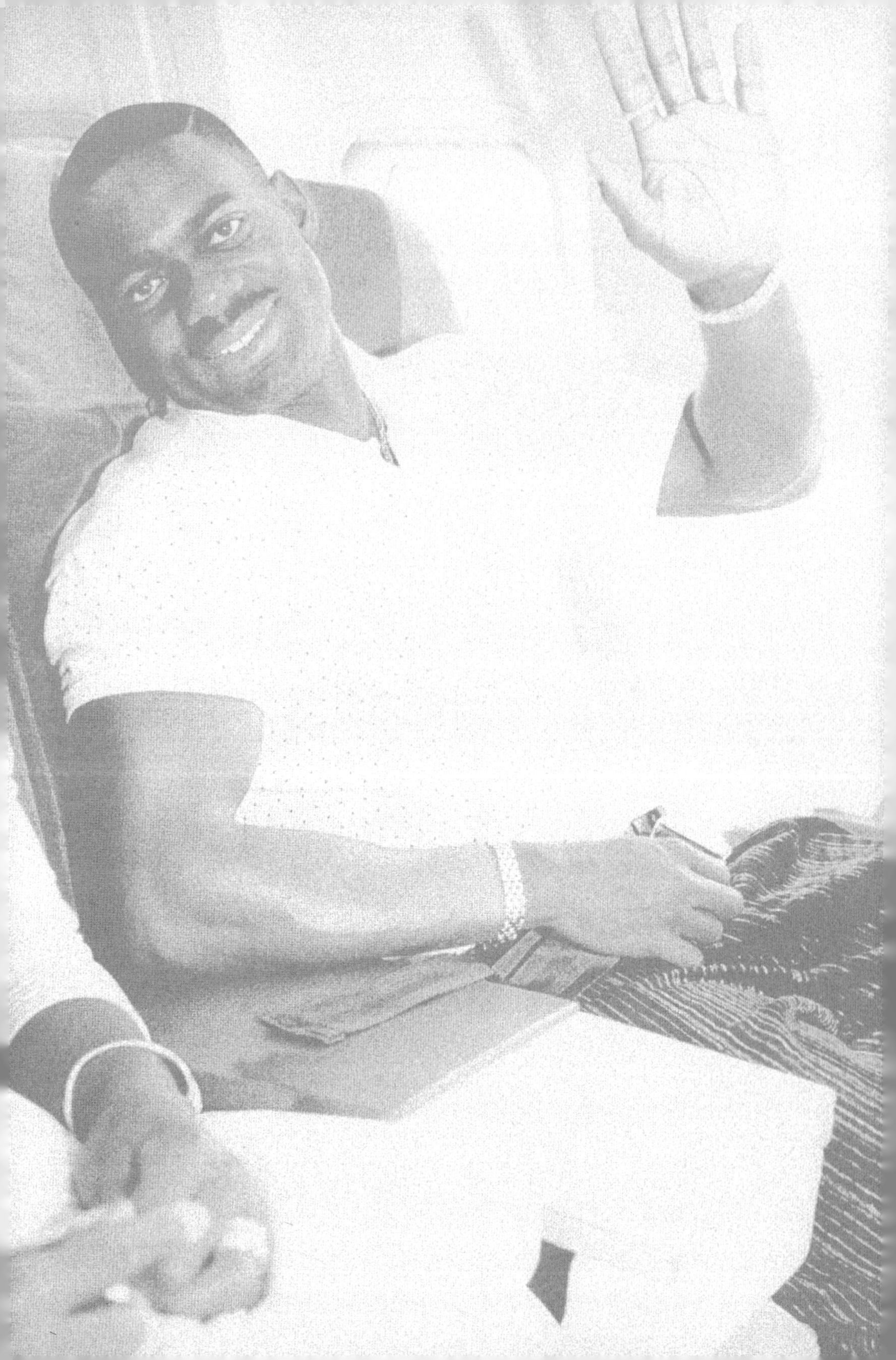

CHAPTER 14

On to Seoul

I returned from St. Kitts, healthy and in time to enter the Canadian National Championships on August 6, 1988. There I served notice: I was back. It had been almost three months since my injury. I was feeling good again. I won the Nationals in 9.90 seconds. I was very glad to be competing again. I performed in a few other meets before going to Italy where in Sestriere, I ran in 9.98 seconds. From there, the team set out for Zürich where Carl and I met for a rematch on August 17, the first time we had competed against each other that season.

Carl won the Zürich race with a time of 9.93. He was ecstatic about his win. He equaled the personal best he achieved in Rome in 1987. His time tied the previous world record, held by Calvin Smith since 1983. I came in third with a time of 10-flat, but I knew I had untapped speed potential. I was content knowing I still had the edge and my hamstring was holding out. It was the first time Carl had beaten me in three years. He went on to declare he would never lose to me again.

Today, it is interesting to reflect on these race times. After the Seoul Olympics when my world record in Rome was disqualified, Carl's time of 9.93 in Zürich 1988 and Rome 1987 became retroactive world records, shared with Calvin Smith. Later, Carl's time of 9.92 in the Seoul 100 metre final also became the new retroactive world record after I was disqualified. In the IAAF World Championships in Tokyo in 1991, Carl ran

9.86, another world record. Carl held the world record from 1987 to 1994, except for two months when Leroy Burrell ran 9.90 in New York in June 1991. My 100 metre time of 9.83 in Rome was not beaten until 1999 by an American, Maurice Greene. My time of 9.79 in Seoul was not beaten until 2002 by another American, Tim Montgomery. Had I not been disqualified in Seoul, and retroactively disqualified in Rome, I would have held the world record for 15 years. But this was not meant to be. I have forgiven everyone and made my peace with the way it all played out.

Needing some time to rest and relax after Zürich, I came home to Toronto for a few days before resuming my preparation for Seoul. Spending time with my mother again was rejuvenating. She prepared some real home cooked meals unlike any I had enjoyed in recent memory.

Meanwhile, I refocused on my program. After our meets in Europe, the Canadian team hosted a training camp in Vancouver, British Columbia. Here, the CTFA selected the athletes who would go to Seoul. While I was in St. Kitts, I gained almost fifteen pounds. A return to full speed sprinting would bring me back to form again. At the next training camp in Tokyo, I continued to work hard.

Our track team gathered in Seoul on September 16, 1988. We were again reminded of our low status. The track team was the last of the Canadian Olympic delegation to leave for Korea. Arriving at the Olympic Village, they discovered the more preferred groups within the Canadian delegation were granted the lower floors while the track team was given the top floor. The complex had only one elevator. When not available, this meant the team had to walk 12 flights down to the lobby. Track athletes do not need to unnecessarily expend precious energy before their races nor potentially risk leg injuries on stairs.

The track team flew in economy class, legs cramped for the duration of the long flight across the Pacific Ocean. In contrast, the shooting team, for example, travelled in first class and arrived early, affording them ample time to rest and adjust to climate and

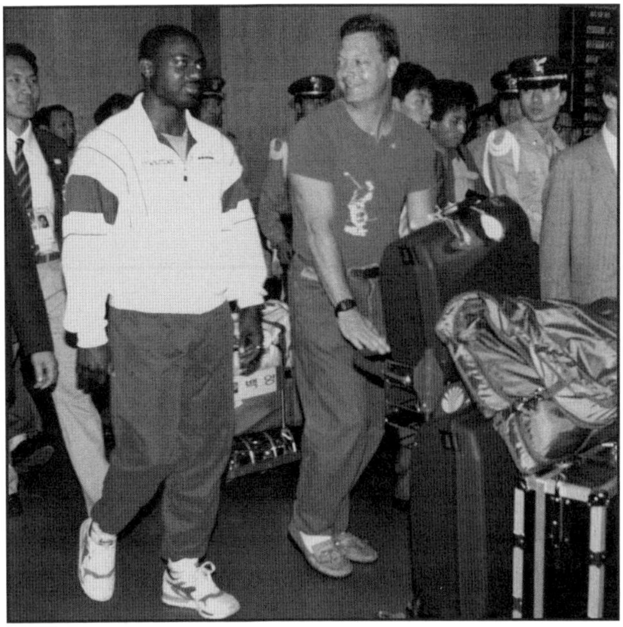

time changes. These biases against Canadian track teams were nothing new to us. They were always a reminder we were never as important as the other Canadian teams. Racial profiling existed at that time and was clearly evident. But today, I can honestly say I have forgiven all.

Compared to the lavishly treated American track team, the Canadian track team felt like second-class citizens. I remember earlier on in my career how American teams would laugh and make jokes about Canadian athletes. We were mocked, our system criticized. We were the laughing stock of the sporting world. Sometimes, team members were embarrassed to wear our Canadian jerseys, afraid of becoming a target for ridicule. I did not share this sentiment. I always wanted to make Canada proud, to make Canada stand out and be respected. And I forgive all those who made fun of us.

Given my past experiences, I chose not to stay in the Olympic Village in Seoul with Charlie and the other members of the track team. The environment within the village was one of sizing up the competition and becoming consumed with who was doing or saying what. All of this was incredibly distracting and decreased my ability to concentrate on the task at hand. Instead, I stayed at the Seoul Hilton. It sounds selfish, but I did not want to be distracted by the chaos. This was a very important race for me. I wanted to stay relaxed and focused.

I also did not attend the opening ceremonies. For this decision, I was criticized heavily. However, the weather in Seoul at the time was extremely hot, sometimes reaching as high as 100 degrees Fahrenheit. I arrived in Korea, only days before my first round of heats. I did not think it was in my best interest to stand in the scorching sun for hours and risk further dehydration. Therefore, while the athletes were parading for hours draining their energy away in the sun, I watched it on television. I was with them in spirit.

Few understood this action on my part. But I knew this was the race of my life, and no matter what anyone thought, I was there to win. It may also sound unfair or unsportsmanlike of me not to join the representatives of my adopted country at the opening ceremonies, but you must appreciate my circumstances. Life had become crazy for me as I was hounded everywhere I went. Between the fans and the media, it was hard to get around peacefully and safely. Even athletes from other countries would ask for my autograph and ask me to pose for pictures. So, in the privacy of my hotel room the days before the heats, I ate, rested and contemplated, mentally preparing myself for the race.

I spent time visualizing myself warming up, running and winning. I would lock this image into my mind and, like stored up energy, release it when the right moment came. Plain and simple, I knew this was the preparation I required to perform as expected. I wanted to win. I knew if I won I would make my family, my training team and my fans very happy. I knew many people around the world wanted to see me win. Really truly in my heart, I did not intend to disappoint anybody. I did not want to let anybody down.

I asked Bryan about these feelings of not wanting to let anyone down. Bryan responded, "Ben, you do not have a master contract that allows you to feel comfortable about being worshipped by anyone. As you describe being famous or those who just look up to you as fans, on your soul this does not sit well with you. Part of the overall experience you went through was to teach the world there is only One God, only One Truth. For you were one of many vessels to show the world that they must not idolize you or worship you or anyone else. For in every case, the ones the world idolizes and worships will fall. Michael Jackson is no different. The lesson for the world: if they want the best for another, do not idolize or worship another."

I said, "Are you saying if the world did not worship me, I would not have fallen?"

Bryan's response was, "Yes. We are all actors on a stage."

Training before the race allowed me to cement in my mind what it was I wanted to achieve. I would meet with the team daily and train with them for about an hour. This does not seem very long, but if I was not ready by now, it was too late. While training was light, I found myself doing my workouts with intensity. Everyone watching my practice expressed amazement at my speed. Yet I remained relaxed. In the weight room, the same thing happened as I went through my routine. All my thoughts were about doing something that had never been done before, doing something special. The words my mother told me many years before resounded in my mind: I was a special boy and here for a purpose. It was clear to me now that this was my purpose and my time. Like a recording in my head, I kept replaying my race in my mind. In each instant, the result was always the same: When the gun go off, the race is over...

Before race day, I did allow myself one act of indiscretion while in Seoul. It was after our last practice. Maybe it was because I was feeling elated about finishing practice, excited now about the upcoming race. While leaving the gym, I ran into Sherri Howard, a member of the US 4 x 100 women's relay team. She was an eye-catcher and a great athlete. Her sister was also on the US team. On seeing her, I immediately went up and started a conversation. I had not gone out socially while in Seoul up until then and had no intentions to go out that night. But for Sherri, I had to make one exception. I invited her out and she accepted. She looked great that night when I met her at about 9 p.m. in the lobby of her hotel where she had been waiting for me. I made sure not to keep her waiting long and was right on time. I was happy to be in her company. The truth was that I had always wanted to go out with her. I had seen her over the years but never really found the nerve to approach her. Now here in Seoul, nerves came easily and so did our conversation over two glasses of champagne. We made a pact not to talk about track and instead talked about family and friends.

We were talking for a while when someone recognized me and beckoned me over to the other side of the restaurant, as if to ask for an autograph. I then got up willingly and went over, leaving my glass unattended. I did not give it much thought at the time. But this was the only time I had anything to drink or eat outside of my hotel room and in the company of anyone else prior to the race. Not wanting to be away from her for too long, I hurried back. When I returned, she appeared uneasy and said her coach had issued a team curfew and she had to leave. We then hastily finished our drinks and left but not before I asked her out again. We exchanged phone numbers. She told me to call her after the Games. I was delighted.

I did not see Sherri after the Games. To this day, I have never heard from her again. On my way back to my hotel, I ran into the fan who had requested my autograph. He inquired if I knew the woman I had been with earlier. I said I knew her, to which he replied, "She is a friend of Carl Lewis. Did you know that?" In fact, I had not known that. Even then, I did not think further about the comment. I was tired and at this point needed to return to rest in the peace and quiet of my hotel room. Before I went to bed, I ordered room service and set about to watch a movie.

Later that night, I received an unexpected phone call from a man who said he was a news reporter from New York. Strict instructions were given to the hotel concierge not to have me disturbed, not even for phone calls. Even my reservation at the hotel was not made under my own name. Only Charlie, Larry, Jamie and my mother knew my room number and were allowed to get through. So, this call was a shock to me. I was puzzled. How did this guy get my phone number? I wondered. In the meantime, the man pestered me with questions: How was I enjoying Seoul? How was I feeling? What kinds of food did I like? Was I dating? I asked him to call back another time.

My food arrived. After I ate, I called my mother and told her what happened. Being a mother, she peppered me with advice. Then she told me of a dream she had. In the dream, I was walking in the country with her. A snake suddenly appeared from under a rock. She was screaming at me to kill the snake. But before I could, it rose up and bit me on the leg. I prayed that night after I hung up. I prayed to God to keep me safe and spare me from anyone who would want to harm me in any way. My understanding at the time was that dreaming of a snake meant encountering an enemy.

I asked Bryan about my mother's dream. God gave me the interpretation:

The snake represents power. It represents revenge against you, Ben. The snake is a symbol of one who will harm you, one who is from Africa. For the snake is from Africa. The snake was there to warn you: The snake bite represented steroids or venom. When a snake bites, it is always selfishly motivated. The snake dream interpreted in its simplest form: you were to be sabotaged by someone planting steroids, only for you to consume.

I know today part of my mother's dream actually did happen. It came to pass. I was, in fact, drugged and sabotaged.

At the practice facility the next morning, there were a lot of people around. Despite the presence of security, I could not trust that I was completely safe from someone wishing to play foul. It was not unusual to run into members of a rival team. Often, this was friendly and sportsmanlike. But at other times, such encounters could become tense and uneasy.

I remember seeing André Jackson. Like Sherri, I had seen him from time to time and he was always friendly. We saw each other in Zürich in 1986 when he mysteriously ended up in the same courtesy car with me, going to the track. Later that evening, we went out to a club together in Zürich. He seemed to come in and out of my life, showing up randomly and each time trying to befriend me. Here in Seoul, he continued to be overly sociable, behaving like we were old friends. Funny enough, he never offered this friendship to others around me and would only show up at times when I was alone. He had come up to me earlier the day before and we chatted for a while as I worked out. André would appear again and again. But I wasn't thinking about André. I was so focused I could allow myself to think of nothing else but race day.

I wanted to win, not so much for myself or to make myself happy, but rather, to make others happy. I got very little joy out of simply winning. My true joy came from seeing others happy and excited because I had won. And so many people wanted to see me win, so many people had come to look up to me. Here I was about to run the race of my life in front of millions of people watching around the whole world. I did not want to let anyone down.

I asked Bryan about this. I asked if God could tell me, why did I feel joy from seeing others happy? How did people view me?

Ben, your master contract was also for people to live their life through you, to find joy through you and also to find hope through you. You lived for others. You did not live for yourself. Joy for you was a far distance away. Many thought that you were a retarded Black man who stutters. For yes, it is true that many close to you took advantage of you in many different ways. The Truth is: You do not have a master contract in this life to be retarded. You have a master contract to only process Truth. Anything that is not of Truth, you do not process easily. This is the same for many who claim to suffer with Attention Deficit Disorder. For these ones are only able to process certain types of Truth. Children with ADD will likely not do well in school, particularly in subjects that are not of Truth. When this happens, they are labeled disabled, just like some have labeled you retarded. You must forgive them all.

I wanted to weep. I did not know any of this. I do forgive them all.

Bryan continued to discern, then added, "For society to get rid of ADD, the school system must teach Truth only. Remember: ADD, even autism, is a barometer that reflects the overall Truth level in a given society. ADD and autism are simply an escape from a world that has mostly accepted untruths and false beliefs."

I did not consciously intend to disappoint anyone in Seoul: my mother, my father, my family, my coaches, my team, my country, my fans, or anyone else. I would not take any chance that would possibly jeopardize this race, a moment we all had been sacrificing for and working toward for so long. Any compromise would only bring extreme pain and suffering to my family and, especially, to my mother. My family is more important to me than winning or being famous. I know sabotage by others was the human cause of me losing my gold medal.

However, I also know the buck stops with me. I am ultimately responsible for losing my gold medal. The bottom line is: Everything was written, based on the experiences I have had from other incarnations, unresolved issues I brought into this life. Knowing this, I have forgiven all. And even more difficult, I have forgiven myself.

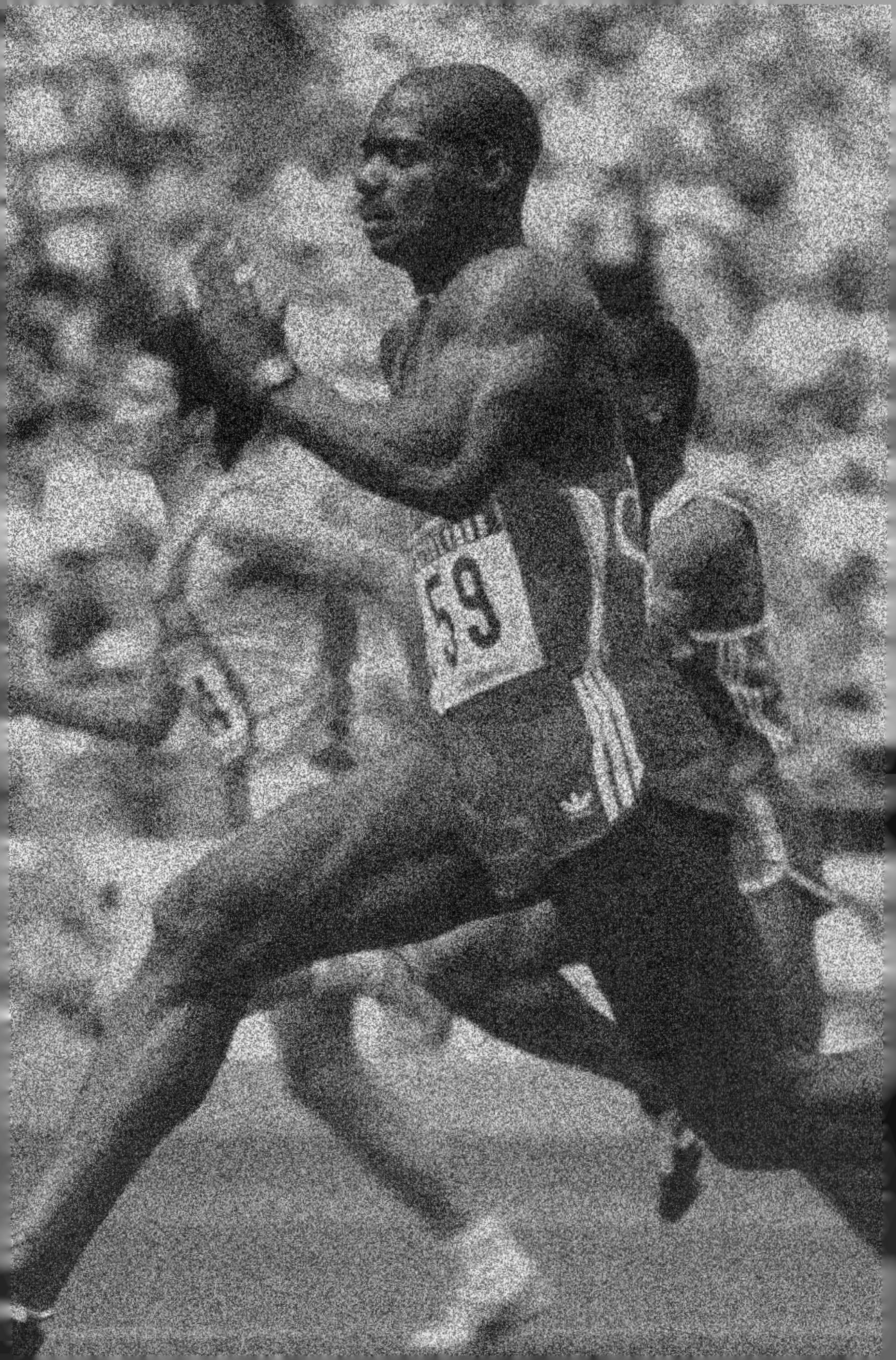
59

CHAPTER 15

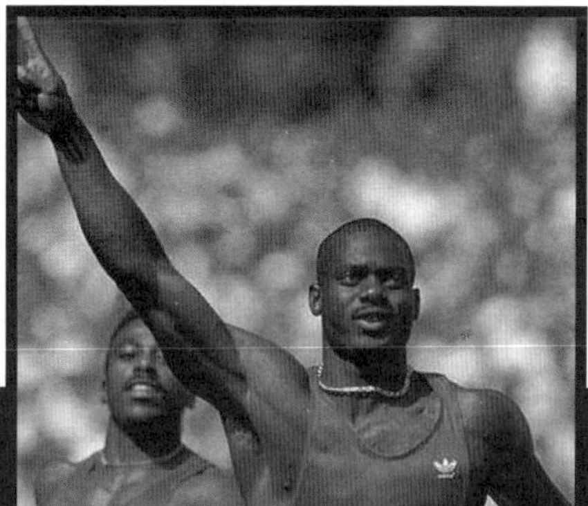

The Chaos of Champions

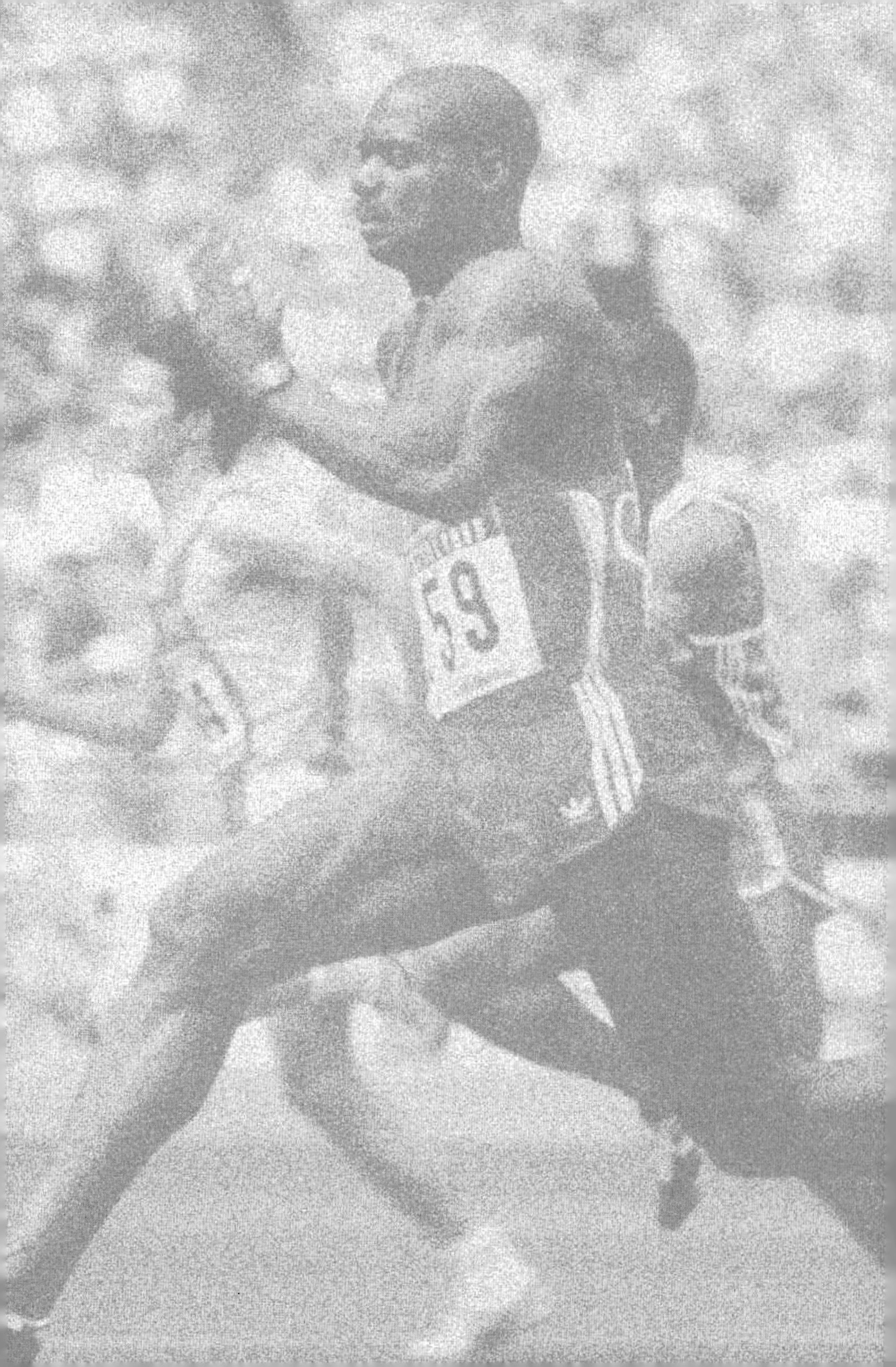
58

CHAPTER 15

The Chaos of Champions

Nothing could penetrate my focus. I was not prepared to allow myself to be distracted. But, I noticed that tension quickly developed between Charlie and Jamie. They argued fiercely, most times out of my earshot. I had my suspicions about what the problem was between them. Jamie wanted compensation. But now was not the time for me to become involved and I knew it. When I first met Jamie, he was neither pushy nor aggressive. But here in Seoul, his behaviour began to concern me, knocking me off centre.

Not understanding or appreciating my need to stay focused, Jamie approached me to discuss compensation. He demanded a million dollars for his services. I was speechless. He continued to be very insistent, although I asked him to defer this discussion until a more appropriate time. He felt Charlie and I were getting all the fame and publicity while he remained in the background. Jamie, no doubt, played a role in my success and deserved some recognition. So, I had no problem rewarding him, but after the Games.

As he was injecting me with cortisone, I told him clearly I was prepared to sign a contract to that effect. I can only assume he did not trust my word. He continued to hound me, wanting his money NOW! With his increasing antagonism and negativity, Jamie was distressing me beyond my limit.

Here I was trying to prepare for one of the most important races of my life and this man seemed to be concerned about one thing and one thing only: his own interest and acknowledgement. Angered, I told him then and there, "When this is over, you are fired!" I had enough of his complaining and his lack of concern for me at this critical time. Jamie then played his blackmail hand, threatening to go public with my steroid protocol if I did not agree to his demands. My anger tripled. At the time, I was disillusioned and disappointed. He has since passed on and I have forgiven him completely for all of this.

I trusted the people around me. I sincerely thought they were looking after my best interests. Moreover, if I succeeded, we all would succeed. Jamie's attitude and demands were truly disappointing to me. We all had our part to play. I was focused on doing my job which was running. Charlie was there to assist me by giving me my training program and workouts. My agent was there to negotiate my contracts and book my engagements. My doctor and my physiotherapist were supposed to keep me healthy and assist me when I was injured. This was the team to support me and enable me to reach my goal.

Where there is money involved, there is often greed and selfish intent. Some members of my team became greedy and lost sight of our mission which was to win. They saw my talent as a vehicle to their own wealth and no longer even seemed to view me as a person. They lost sight of my needs and my interests and they lost sight of me.

I was brought up in a good family with strong spiritual values. I asked Bryan, "What does it mean to have strong spiritual values?"

Bryan replied, "Ben, for one to be truly spiritual, one must be able to love oneself and love others unconditionally. And one must be able to forgive oneself and others unconditionally. For if one is not able to do this, and one claims to belong to a religion, this one has given their power away. This one feels unworthy. This one refuses to take self-accountability and self-responsibility. This one, in most cases, refuses to believe in past lives. For this one does not wish to revisit the past life of guilt, shame, anger, fear or whatever it is. They do not wish to confront it. Just like you received a miracle healing and your depression was lifted, if we did not go into your past life, that would not have been lifted. To be spiritual is to know Truth, is to know God. To be religious is to walk through the potential trap door of false beliefs. From one life to the next, you remain on this treadmill of suffering."

In my relationships and my track life, I have tried to focus on good things, staying positive, being respectful to people, not being mean-spirited and avoiding trouble. My mother, who was my confidante, instilled in me a gentle spirit. I trusted her and her judgment. She was a strong woman. I respected her for that. She lived her life with great courage. While going through my own ordeals and trials, I drew from her courage. It is this courage that has always kept me going. It was this courage that picked me up in the middle of the mayhem that was Seoul.

I asked Bryan about the courage that came from my mother. I asked him to discern if this was true. God clarified it for me:

Ben, you ask another question about courage, if your courage came from your mother. Your courage did come from your mother, through a belief system. Your mother gave you three beliefs that gave you courage. The first belief she gave you was that you can achieve anything if you work hard. And this is what you did throughout your journey. Secondly, she gave you a belief, a strong belief, that you are a failure only if you give up. For throughout your journey, you have always been determined not to give up. And thirdly, she gave you a very powerful belief that you are always worthy of success, that you are always worthy. These are the three beliefs that your mother gave you.

But I say to you and all My Children: there is another belief that gives you much greater courage. That is the belief, the knowing that I am a loving God and that I am always there for you, for My Children.

At the Olympics, the 100 metre race is a highlight, a centerpiece of the Games. For me personally, everything was tied to this one race, an event that could last less than ten seconds. For me, it was about not letting anyone down, from my mother to my coach and entourage, to my sponsors, to my country. With almost the whole world watching, I knew the stakes were high.

My mother and sister were in Seoul to watch. Dad was held up in Jamaica due to a hurricane. Jamaica had suffered significantly as a result of Hurricane Gilbert. The Island was devastated and no flights were allowed in or out of the airport. Even to this day, the residents of Jamaica still talk about Gilbert, the worst storm to ever hit the Island. But no doubt, Dad would be watching on television. Knowing my parents were there to support me and my dream spurred me on.

There were four rounds held over a period of two days before the ultimate moment, the final race. The Olympics, with its many preliminaries, can be grueling. The objective is to make it through the heats and still have enough energy reserved in the tank to go all out for victory in the finals. Palms are clammy. Shirts are soaked in nervous sweat. Approximately 100 runners get ready to battle it out in 13 heats. In the end, only eight of us will make it to the final race. Only one of us will win. There are no draws. No extra time or overtime. No second chances. There can only be one winner. Every runner worth his salt thinks it is going to be him.

Everyone there had made it because they considered themselves to be champions. To varying degrees, we all postured, posed and strutted, trying to look cool, psyche out and intimidate the guy next door. But in the end, what mattered most was who could get across the finish line first. And that day, in the silence of my consciousness, I knew I was ready. "I will be the one," I said to myself. Whether it was a sore hamstring, stiff quads or a hurting Achilles, my aches and pains would have to wait. For when the gun go off, I'll be gone...

Some have called what followed in Seoul one of the biggest sports stories of our time. It seems like everyone remembers the final in Seoul. But I also ran two beautiful heats and a semifinal at those Games, races you probably have never heard about, especially if you have never followed the sport before. I say these races were beautiful, not out of arrogance. It was wonderful for me to have come this far, to be here after so much and with so little.

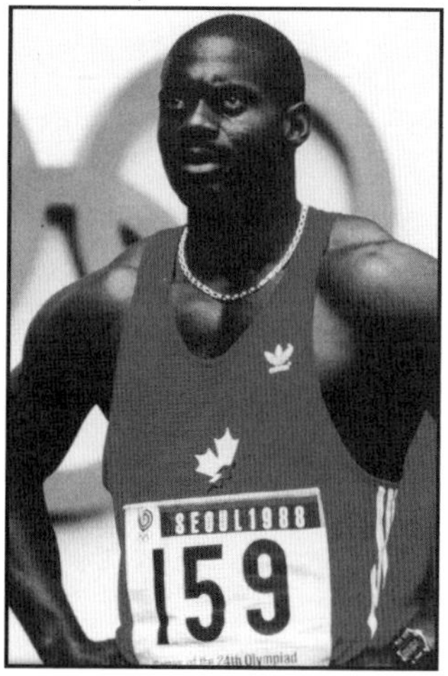

From the possibility of death as an infant, I had overcome so much to be here now. I was ready to run the first heat in the 100 metres for Canada in the Games of the XXIV Olympiad... that was something beautiful. Dressed in my black and gold Diadora running shoes and decked out with a gold chain around my neck, I kneeled in my stance the way I have always done, gave thanks to God and spread my hands out across the width of my lane. I was coiled and ready to go. And at the crack of the gun, "go" I did. The first heat left no doubt. At 60 metres I was so far ahead I could virtually coast to victory. Once I realized I was in the lead, I began decelerating so as to save my effort for later. The crowd laughed.

The second heat two hours later would be more challenging. With only the top two finishers moving on to the semifinals, it was important to nip this race, especially now that I was up against two stellar contenders: Linford Christie and Dennis Mitchell. I also knew that the four runners with the best overall time would be allowed through to the semifinals. But even so, I could not take too many chances with these two competitors.

Meanwhile, Carl Lewis had established himself in his heats by running quick times early. It seemed his strategy was to intimidate. For now, I simply wanted to coast through and reserve my energy for the right time. But with Christie and Mitchell, how much coasting could I do without being eliminated?

This is why this second heat was beautiful: I came in third and still made it! I had taken off without hesitation and had taken a sizeable lead by the 60-metre mark when I slowed down once again to conserve my energy. The crowd went wild. They must have thought I had made a tactical mistake. Some thought I was hurt but I was not. It seemed I had shut down too early and I had not performed well enough to make it to the semifinals. Christie won in 10.11, Mitchell came second in 10.13, while I made it in quietly in 10.17.

Many people, including Charlie, thought I probably would not make it through as a result of my apparent miscalculation. Nerves were worked up and my coaching team was worried. Would I make it or not? "What the hell are you doing? That time may not be good enough to make it through to the semifinal!" Charlie exclaimed when he came over to me. We would have to wait for five other heats to find out. We watched the rest of the remaining heats in silence, anxiously waiting. Sure enough, none of the remaining heats were fast enough to knock me out of the semifinals. Phew! When it was over, I assured Charlie I would not fool around in the semifinals and I would turn on all 36 valves. Charlie was pleased.

I asked Bryan to ask God, "Why did I not run as fast in the second heat?"

Ben, you ask the question, why did you not run as fast in the second heat? Ben, you must go back to that moment. You were very cocky and you were too sure of yourself, and you under-estimated the other runners. You did not run using the fuel of fear.

I asked Bryan about Charlie's reaction to my second heat. He closed his eyes and he started to discern. As he opened his eyes, Bryan responded to me, "Ben, despite what Charlie Francis said to you or to others, he always believed in your ability. He had no doubt you would make the finals in Seoul. But Charlie did have three worries about you in Seoul, prior to you being awarded the gold medal. He felt you were stubborn at times and would not listen to his instructions. You trusted, at times, the wrong people and he could not be with you 24 hours. His third worry was a deep personal worry: After winning the gold medal, he thought you would be taken away by others, and you would forget about him.

"Remember the first time you ever met Charlie Francis? The first time your eyes connected with Charlie's? Let me remind you about your thoughts of Charlie in the first

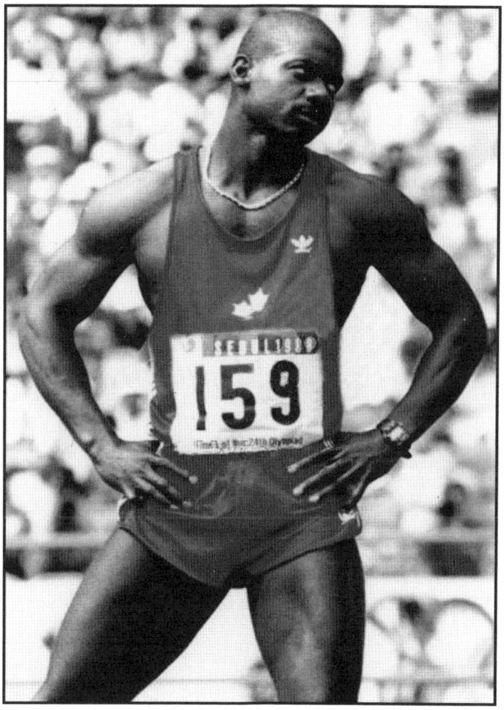

hour. Remember, you only had a 50% comfort level with Charlie? How can this be? Again, allow me to remind you. You only had two dominant thoughts about him. The first thought was clear: You were wondering if you were good enough for Charlie. Now, allow me to remind you of the second: You believed Charlie was a no-nonsense type of man. To you, within the first hour of setting eyes on Charlie Francis, this is how you summed him up. What do you think of what I've just said?"

I said, "Bryan, how do you know so much?"

Bryan's response was, "It is God who works through me. My physical body is just the shell. But what I'm saying to you, is it true?" I responded that it was. That's exactly how I felt about Charlie.

September 24, 1988 was a beautiful day. I got up early to a clear sky. The sun was out. As I looked up from my balcony that morning, I prayed. I asked for protection and guidance. I also asked that God's Will be done, knowing whether I won the gold or not, I would still be happy in God's Hands.

Over 11 years of training, constant pressure and pounding had injured my Achilles tendon. In 1988, it flared up, becoming inflamed and very sore as a result of my intense training for Seoul. By September, my heel was still sore. I would soon be in Waldemar's hands for treatment. But I could not worry about that right now. I had a semifinal to run. Christie and Mitchell would be in my heat once again, with five others. Lewis in his semifinal had a false start before getting it right the second time to win his race in 9.97 seconds.

Stepping up and performing under these nail-biting circumstances was the motivation I needed to win. As I settled into the blocks, I tuned out everything around me. I was ready. The gun then went off and I reacted. I was well on my way when I heard the gun a second time. I turned around to see an official walking toward my lane. They said the false start was mine. I knew my reaction was perfect. Others knew it, too. The crowd booed. Charlie was on his feet. Angry, I told the starter, "That was not a false start! Are you upset that I was able to beat your gun?" Putting him out of my mind, I returned to my position behind the blocks to calm down and reset. As I prepared and crouched in the blocks, I decided not to hold anything back. But I knew I had to be cautious. I knew I had to be aggressive, but not too aggressive. A second false start would disqualify me. When the gun barked again, I paused a little, then took off like a rocket, but with no less force than before. This time, I was in the lead from the very beginning.

I bolted like there was no tomorrow. At about 40 metres down, I went into overdrive. By 80 metres, I realized I could just coast across the finish line, coming in with a time of 10.03 seconds into a headwind. I felt somewhat vindicated later when officials announced that my false start was their mistake. On reviewing the tape, they discovered on coming out of the blocks, I had broken the sensor. Puzzled and unsure what to do, the official incorrectly charged me with a false start. I was happy when they reversed their decision. But I still did not trust the starter's judgment, especially now when I was about to run a final where my quick-edged start would be important. It would be two and a half hours before my showdown with destiny.

I asked Bryan to discern whether or not I truly did have a false start. I watched Bryan close his eyes as he communicated with God. He came back with the answer, "God confirms, in this instance, you did not have a false start. You were falsely accused and you must forgive them." I do forgive them.

After the semifinal, I jogged down and went to the Canadian athletes' tent located at the end of the field. I lay down to rest for awhile, only to be awakened by André Jackson, who wanted to wish me success in the finals. Soon, I could hear the announcer's voice calling for the men's 100 metre finals. It was the finals first call to report to the check-in area. I still wanted to rest and so I laid back down, telling Desai who was in the tent with me not to worry, that we had more than enough time. In what seemed like only seconds, the second call to report went out, and from the tent I could see Lindford Christie and Carl Lewis already out on the track warming up. The heat out there was intense.

I wanted to get as much rest as possible and avoid the extreme temperature out on the track. I was still resting when the third and final call was issued, at which point I knew I had to get up. I sat up. I put my running shoes back on and emerged out onto the warm-up track. I jogged a lap and then stretched. I then replaced my running shoes with my spikes before doing a few warm-up starts out of the blocks. I was the last to reach the calling room but now I was ready.

When I lined up in my lane, I was prepared to show the world something they had never seen before. I positioned myself in the blocks and focused on my dream... my dream to win and bring joy to the hearts of many. The second I got out of the blocks at the final of the 100 metres at Seoul, I knew the race was mine. At no time between hearing the starter's pistol and crossing the finish line did I feel like I could lose that race. I was first out of the blocks. I was leading at 60 metres and no one in the field was strong enough to catch me. At 80 metres, I knew it was a world record run. I just knew it. My endurance was there. I was maintaining my speed and my form.

The race was over. Many in the stadium were filled with great enthusiasm and joy, screaming and waving Canadian flags. I guess I was the sentimental favourite, if not the outright favourite. People wanted me to win and they were happy I had won. I had won the gold medal in the 100 metre dash at the Olympic Games, in 9.79 seconds. I was the Olympic Champion. And with the World Championship I won in Rome the year before, and the world record I set then, 9.83, there was no dispute: I was now the fastest man on Earth.

Winning this race was what drove me to train and push myself beyond human limits for more than 11 years. But before I even looked at the clock to see my time, I was thinking about winning again. I was focused on the fact that I would run faster the next chance I got. I knew if I pushed myself, I could go even faster.

So many things have been said and written about that final race:

Unbelievable... incredible... absolutely incredible... The waiting is over and the question has been answered... We have a new world record... This was the best start of Ben Johnson's life... He did far better than he did in Rome... Here is a man who did what he said he would do... He has set a new standard in starts... His reaction time is the best there is... He looks now to be much faster than Carl has ever been... I think Carl Lewis was flabbergasted... Johnson has silenced his critics...

But the stories did not end there:

On a sunlit September afternoon in 1988 Ben Johnson stepped up to his blocks to run the most important race of his life: the Olympic 100 metres final... Johnson symbolized the Canadian dream–the shy immigrant from Jamaica whose genius was discovered on the frozen running tracks of

> Canada... Johnson ran on talent but he also ran on a lie... For years he had used steroids to boost his performance... And in 46 strides he guaranteed himself sporting immortality by running faster than any man in history... Two days later Johnson was at the center of the biggest scandal in the modern Olympiad... This is the story of how an anabolic steroid called stanozolol blew open the biggest conspiracy of silence in the history of sports and how a lie ruined Ben Johnson's life...

As I reflect on the things the media said about me, I must agree that some things are true. But one thing is definitely not true: My life was never ruined. I knew all was not lost when I returned to Toronto. Camped outside on the front lawn of my home was a crowd of people holding signs saying: We Still Believe in You Ben, We Love You Ben, Show Them They are Wrong. I very much appreciated this kind of public support from fans. And with support from my family, I knew I would not give up. I knew my life would go on. And it did.

There is more to my story than steroid use. There is more to my story than a sabotaged gold medal race. Lost in the scandal is the beauty of triumph that I experienced. On September 24, 1988 the world witnessed the fastest race ever. What I was able to achieve on the track in Seoul was an incredible athletic achievement. I was born to run. And I love to run.

The truth I live with is that I did win that gold medal. On an intuitive level, many in the world know this is true. They know I was cheated out of that medal. The world must remember... if I had taken steroids on the day of the race, these steroids would have seriously hampered my ability to sprint. With stanozolol in my system, it would not have been physically possible for me or anyone else to run a time of 9.79. If I had done this, I never could have won the gold medal.

Years later, while reflecting on Seoul with Bryan, I asked him, "Was this all worth it?" Bryan looked at me with a calmness that comes over him. "Ben, Michael Jackson was known as the King of Pop. Elvis Presley was the King of Rock and Roll. Muhammad Ali was known as the Greatest. You believed you were the King of Sprints. Look what has happened to you and the others. Do you think it's wise for Wayne Gretzky to want to be known as the Great One? Do you think it's wise for Donald Trump to want to be known as the King of the Deal, or for Carl Lewis to want to be known as King Carl? Is it wise for anyone to try to be more famous than God?"

I said to him, "The God Who works through you is wise. From this moment on, I will not look at myself as being better than another. Father, please forgive me."

Bryan closed his eyes and discerned. When he opened his eyes, he informed me, "The records in God's Archives now show that your forgiveness has been accepted and you have been forgiven."

The last 22 years have given me time to reflect on my life and running career. Looking back now, I realize that at times, I had a strong desire to be worshipped. I have often wondered where this desire came from. How did I fall into this trap? I had mixed feelings: There were times when I wanted to be worshipped and there were times when I definitely did not. I did not understand where this could be coming from. My experiences with Bryan have shown me there is almost always a deeper explanation to just about everything.

I asked Bryan to discern whatever Truth it was that I needed to know. I surrendered to the process and prepared myself, knowing by now, I could very well be surprised by an unexpected answer. So, I asked him to ask God, "Where did I ever get this desire to be worshipped?"

Ben, for you ask a question that cannot be answered to your complete satisfaction. For there is so much more that you need to understand. And as you go on your spiritual journey, as you seek Me out, understanding will come. Your soul exists in layers. Your main soul: that is for this life experience. And the other layers of soul, of souls... for you have many, for you've had many different life experiences, not just one... for each other life experience can be called a fractured soul: that is attached to your current life soul. And in most cases, it is the fractured soul that causes you to experience that which is required to fulfill your continuous sowing and reaping contracts.

Ben, you do have a fractured soul that has three false beliefs that have influenced you greatly in this life, stemming from a life where you were known as Khufu in the Ancient Egyptian times. For you believed at that time: If you are not God, you are not worthy. You believed: If you are not God, you do not deserve to live. And you believed: If you are God, you are untouchable.

For this will be removed from you. These false beliefs will be removed from you, as they have carried with you forward into subsequent life experiences, other incarnations, from when you were Khufu, to this time now. For your current soul does not possess these beliefs. This is why you at times experience mixed feelings about whether or not you wish to be worshipped, you wish to be God.

In my silence, away from the noise, I know my true worth. I realize my life experience was designed to teach me spiritual lessons. I know now that one must not take on the role of God or be idolized or worshipped by others. If there is a message from my life that I can share with others, it is this: Great things happen when you surrender to Truth.

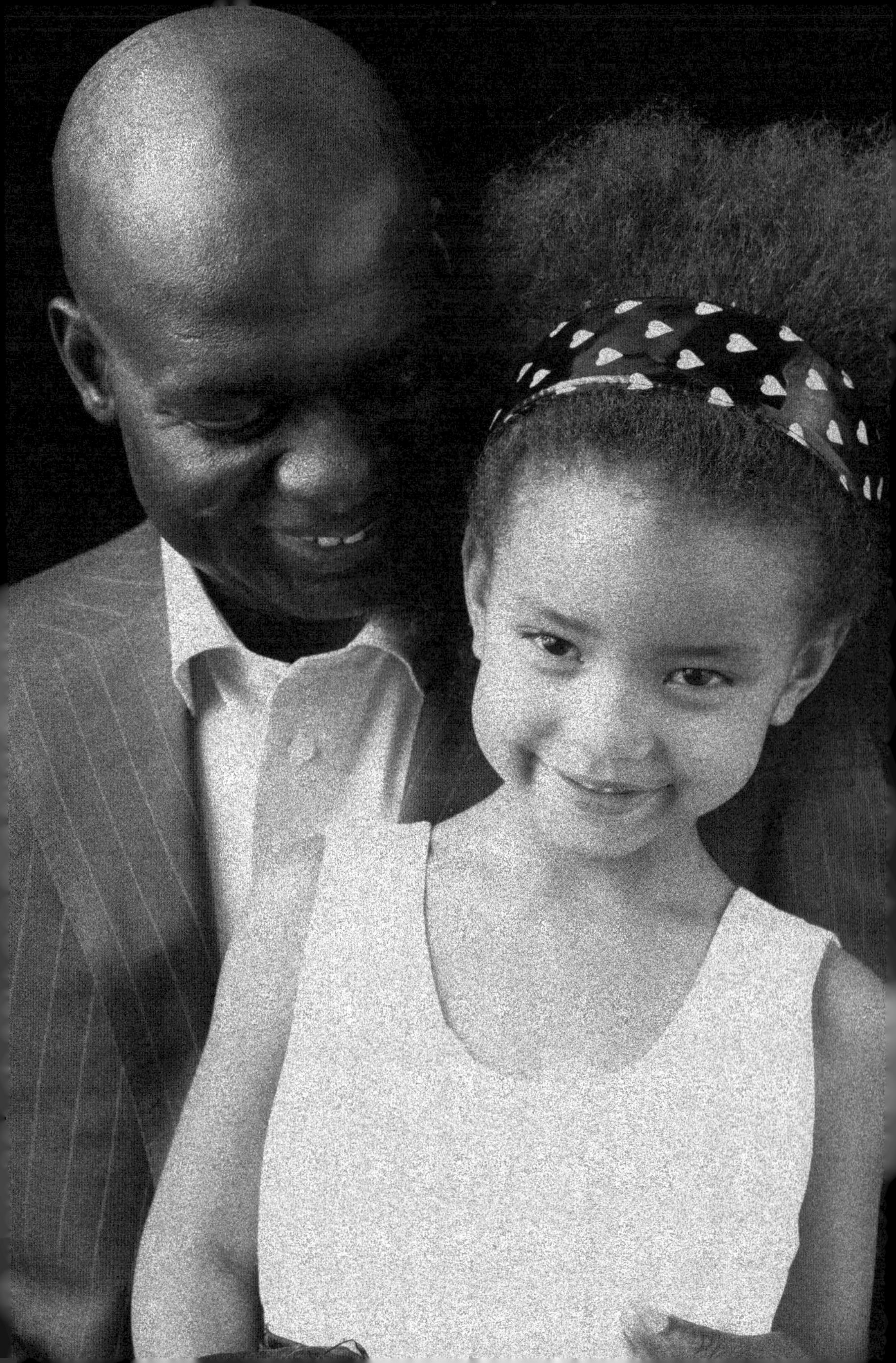

CHAPTER 16

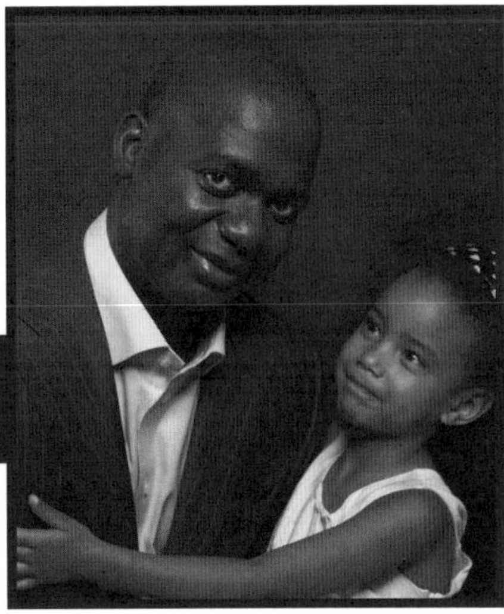

Life after Seoul

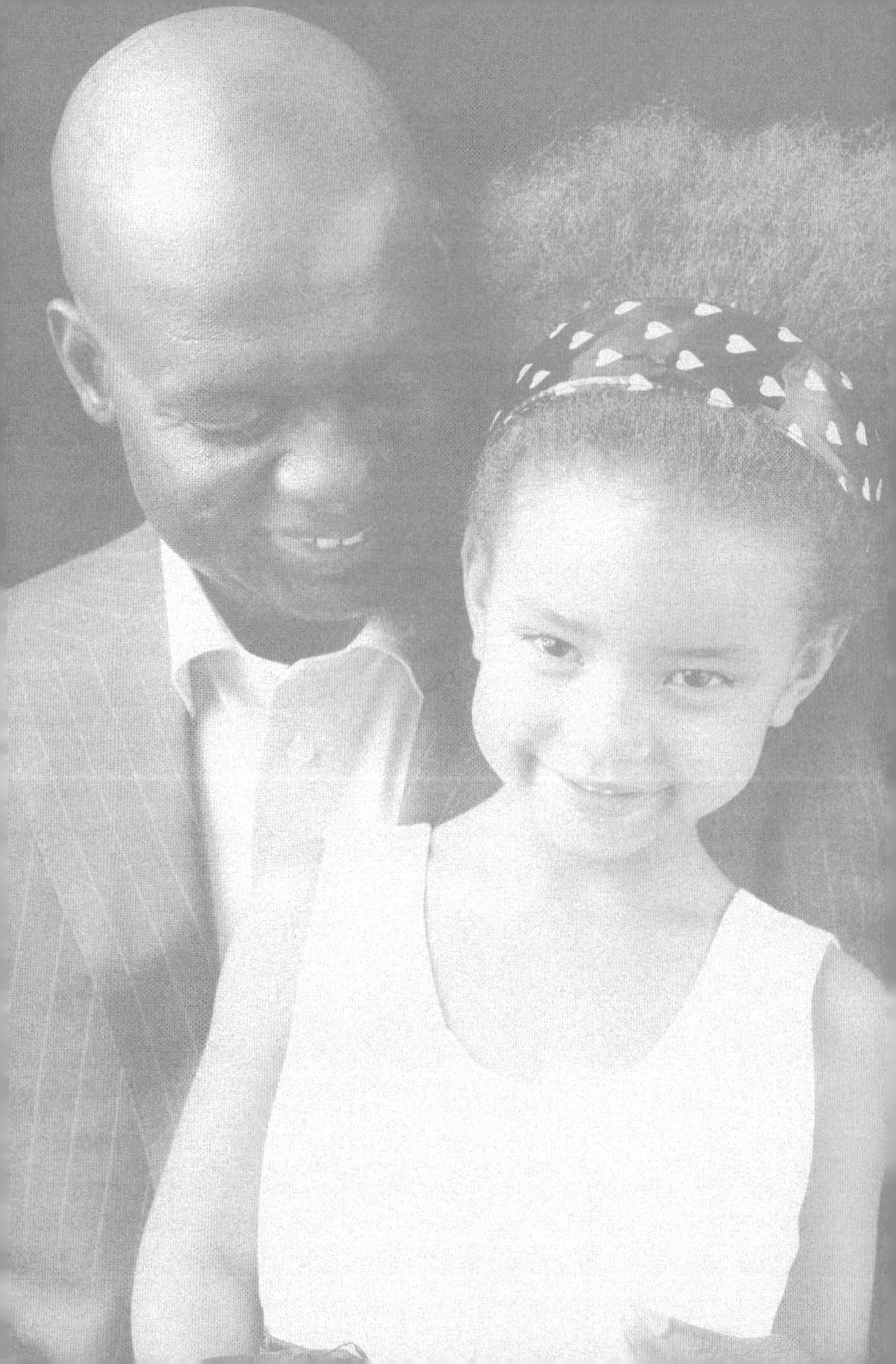

CHAPTER 16

Life After Seoul

I enjoy coaching. Through this means, I am able to share with young athletes the best of my knowledge and, hopefully, give them the benefit of my experience. I tell them to believe in themselves and to choose their friends carefully. I motivate them to make good decisions about how to treat their bodies.

Based on my experience in Seoul, if I were asked, I would suggest to kids and everyone else to learn from my experience: Do not take steroids in the first place. I should have gone with my own original intuition, which God gave me, and trusted in my inner self only. I should not have trusted in man.

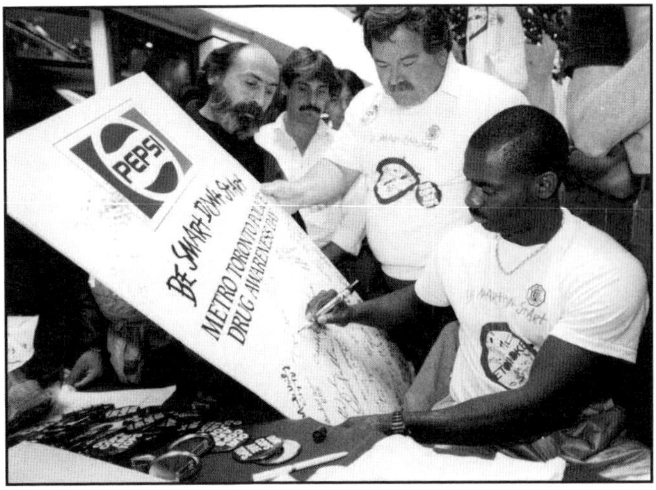

I advise the athletes I train to maintain their determination and stay motivated despite setbacks and disappointments. I urge them to pursue an education. I explain that money is not everything. But when someone has money, he or she should manage it carefully and consider helping those less fortunate. I teach them to conserve their energy, practice regularly, discipline themselves, and develop a strong and loving heart. Most of all, I encourage young people and athletes, when they win, to give God all the glory. I did not always do this throughout my career. I found that placing God front and centre in my life is the best way to go.

It is through helping others that I have found the most fulfillment. I know I have had, and will continue to have, some kind of significant influence on others. Very early on in my career, I recognized the importance of being a role model. I will never forget the first time I signed an autograph. It was at the Junior Championships in Sudbury held in 1980. I was returning to the dressing room when a little boy ran up to me shouting out my name. He was extremely excited. I did not know what to do. Charlie, witnessing what was happening, shouted at me to stop. I looked down to see a child who was beside himself with glee. As I approached him, he was so thrilled he was clearly unable to contain himself. Laughing, almost uncontrollably, he asked for my autograph. It was a happy moment for me to see the joy in this child's eyes. I asked him his name and signed the program he had in his hand. His happiness was evident and the look on his face was something that I had never seen before, nor will I ever forget. It was pleasing to me. It was a most enjoyable experience to be able to give back to this child.

Until then, I had no idea that I could have made someone this happy by simply signing an autograph. The boy took his dad's hand and cheerfully walked away like he was on cloud nine. But as I stood there watching them walk away, it was my turn to admire this boy and his father. Charlie told me afterwards the father had taken time off from work so he could take his son to come and see me run. I was truly amazed someone would go to that extent to see me do something I love to do, especially a father and son enjoying time together. Over the length of my career, I have been touched like this many times. That is the reason I try to give back whenever I can.

I enjoy charity work. I volunteered for a couple of years with a group of school dropouts. A teacher approached me asking if I could assist her with the students. I agreed. These kids all had dreams of making it to the NBA or NFL and thought they did not need a formal education. Although I am convinced you have to believe in your dreams, I knew from personal experience that you also need a strong foundation to be able to reach them. An abandoned building the teacher wanted to use for this purpose needed funding in order to repair it. The government had planned to demolish the building. But when the teacher applied for funding and described the curriculum, the government agreed to support the program. I was very happy when she told me her request had been approved.

About a month later, the funding came through. For three days per week I worked with her, motivating the children to go back to school. Over time, there was remarkable improvement among the students. Some have even gone on to higher learning. It was amazing to see and to be a part of such a worthwhile and successful program.

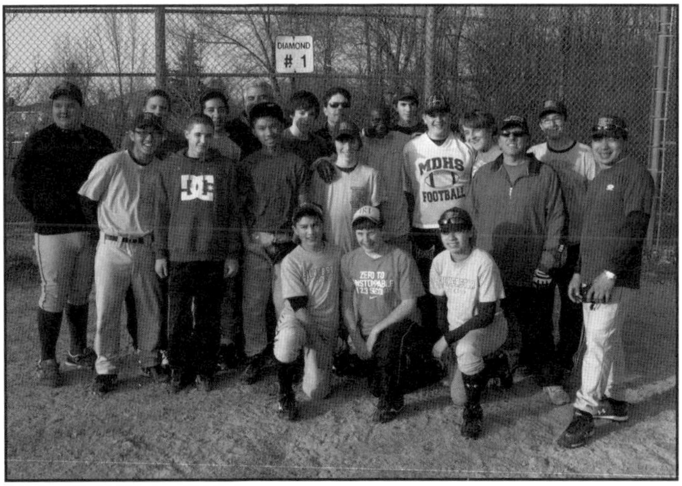

Speaking to Bryan one day, I was amazed to learn school dropouts are actually spiritually-driven kids who have been misguided. Many will have apparent symptoms of ADD. Most children with ADD don't need a drug: They just need Truth. I asked Bryan to explain more. Why do so many of these kids drop out? As usual, immediately after I asked, Bryan closed his eyes as he always does when he communicates with the Heavens. Then the information simply flows out. Sometimes, Bryan will abruptly stop talking and just close his eyes again to receive more information. It truly is amazing how he is able to confirm God's Truth.

After Bryan opened his eyes, he began to answer my question. "Ben, most children who drop out of school have three separate master programs or master contracts that influence their behaviour, which over time, may cause them to drop out of school prematurely. The first key master program is the fact that these children, young adults have never been able to overcome rejection. The inability to overcome rejection is the fuel for their anger. The second master program most of these school dropouts have is their inability to understand man's logic. When I say logic, I mean man's understanding of what truth is. Ironically, they reject man's truth and are desperately seeking God's Truth. Instead of man's logic, many of these dropouts prefer a world of fantasy. It is less painful. The third master program that is common in most of these school dropouts is their inability to cope with certain types of fear. Their most common fear is fear of failure. So they avoid success, hoping they will not have to experience some level of failure resulting from that success. They also fear persecution for believing God's Truth, based on past life experiences of taking a spiritual path. There are no other reasons to focus on, explaining why many of these individuals drop out of school.

"Ben, you are attracted to helping these individuals: Just like they dropped out of school, so did you. You are attracted to helping these individuals who are the mirror of you, on some level. Both sides are only searching for the answer to the question: Why?

"And Ben, please notice: this response, as I have received it from the Heavens, did not require a feasibility study costing $1 million. The information has been given to you freely. And I say unto you, Ben, even if you were to spend $1 billion, would anyone come up with the same answer?"

I replied, "No."

Bryan then asked me, "How do you know?"

And I said, "After the healing I have received from my symptoms of depression and the heavy weight on my head, I just know. I am now able to be more accepting of God's Truth when I hear it."

On another occasion, I received a letter from a social worker who wanted my help. She was counseling a fourteen-year-old boy whose father had recently died. It was a week before Christmas and the boy was angry at the world for taking his father away from him. He refused to communicate with anyone. The social worker, in an effort to take the boy out of his grief, asked him what he wanted for Christmas. He requested a poster of me. He said I had a lot of bad things happen to me and because of this I would understand what he was going through. He was looking for a friend in me.

I read the letter and thought about this boy's situation a lot before calling the social worker. I told her I wanted to deliver the poster personally. Two days before Christmas, the social worker and I went to the boy's house. He and I talked. Through tears, he told me how his dad died. I listened and saw myself in him. I told him to live his life in a way that would make his dad proud. Then I gave him the poster and signed it for him. A month later, the social worker called saying the boy had improved dramatically since he met me. Again, I found it remarkable that in one visit and just a short chat, I could have changed someone's life for the better. I am so glad I took the time to help.

I share these experiences not to boast. I have nothing to boast about except having had a chance to make others happy. But after Seoul, some thought my life had ended. In fact, my life simply changed gears, switched tracks. I took on a new purpose.

In 1990, I appeared as a guest on a television show called the Neon Rider. A Canadian drama series, the show was about a man who had quit his job to become a mentor to troubled teens. He would take the teens to his ranch where he would teach them about life. I often watched the show and was pleased to have been invited to appear on it. My acting role was to be a guest at the ranch and mentor a young boy who had been disfigured in a fire. During my track career, there were many things I was prohibited from doing for fear of being injured. One of those was horseback riding. I had never been on horseback. With my two-year suspension and my track career on hold, I was now free to experience and do many things I had never had the opportunity to do before. I have always loved the outdoors and horses, not to mention Western movies, so I was pleased to have had this chance of a lifetime.

After Seoul, I traveled to places I had never been before. Although I had travelled extensively during my running career, the only places I had visited were those that had track and field competitions. Now I was being invited to different engagements and venues. I was on a different circuit now, meeting and speaking to people who may not have been track and field fans.

After all these years, I am still encouraged by the fact that many of my fans remain non-judgmental. At a recent interview I gave in Toronto, the journalist, who was from Europe, could not believe how many people came up to me to say hello and shake my hand. I told him this was an everyday occurrence that has become a part of my life. Surprised by this, he said it was a measure of true success that people still regarded me with so much respect. I thank him for the compliment.

Through all the difficult times I faced in my life, my famiily has always stood by me and I thank God for them. Without their love and support, I don't know how I would have made it to this day. In 1990, I lost my father. He had been with me from afar in spirit throughout my career and the whole turmoil of events post Seoul. I spoke to him often. He started to make plans to come and join us in Canada after his retirement. But sadly, before this could happen, he suffered a massive and fatal stroke. His plan to come to Canada was not to be. Losing my parents was much more difficult than anything I ever had to face during or after my track career.

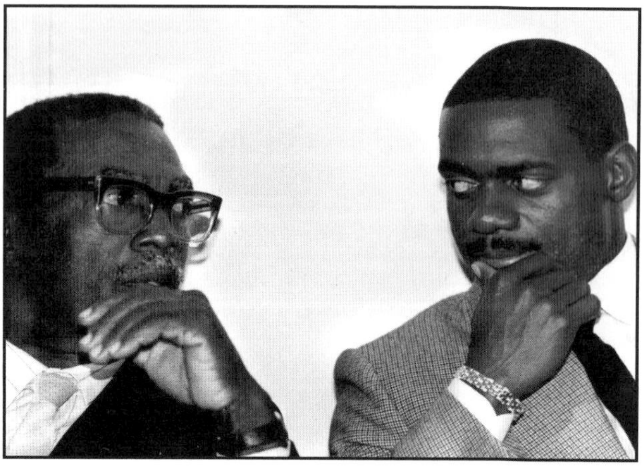

When all is said and done, one of my biggest accomplishments has nothing to do with my career. My biggest achievement happened when I became a father. I have kept this part of my life protected from public view until now. I had a daughter out of wedlock and I thank God for her. I also thank Sharon, her mother, for this beautiful girl. Her name is Jeneil Johnson. She in turn has given birth to my precious granddaughter with the sweet name of Micaila Valerie Johnson. They are my biggest pride and joy.

Micaila, who is now five, loves to play sports. Already she shows a love for running. When possible, I take her out with me to the track. Much to my amusement, Micaila also loves to sing and dance. Just the other day, she was singing to me as I was driving with her in the car. She was singing the reggae classic, Three Little Birds by Bob Marley: "Don't worry 'bout a ting... 'Cause every little ting gonna be alright..." I asked her if I could sing along with her. At first, she agreed. But shortly after I started to sing with her, she said in a very matter-of-fact way, "No, Grandpa, you don't know the song... Only I should sing!" And she just carried on singing, as I continued to drive, hiding my amusement. One thing I love and admire about Micaila: My sweet little granddaughter has no problem speaking her mind! My daughter, Jeneil, who also loved to run track, has recently taken an interest in law. I am proud to report that she is currently attending community college to further her education. It is rewarding to see the next generations carrying on.

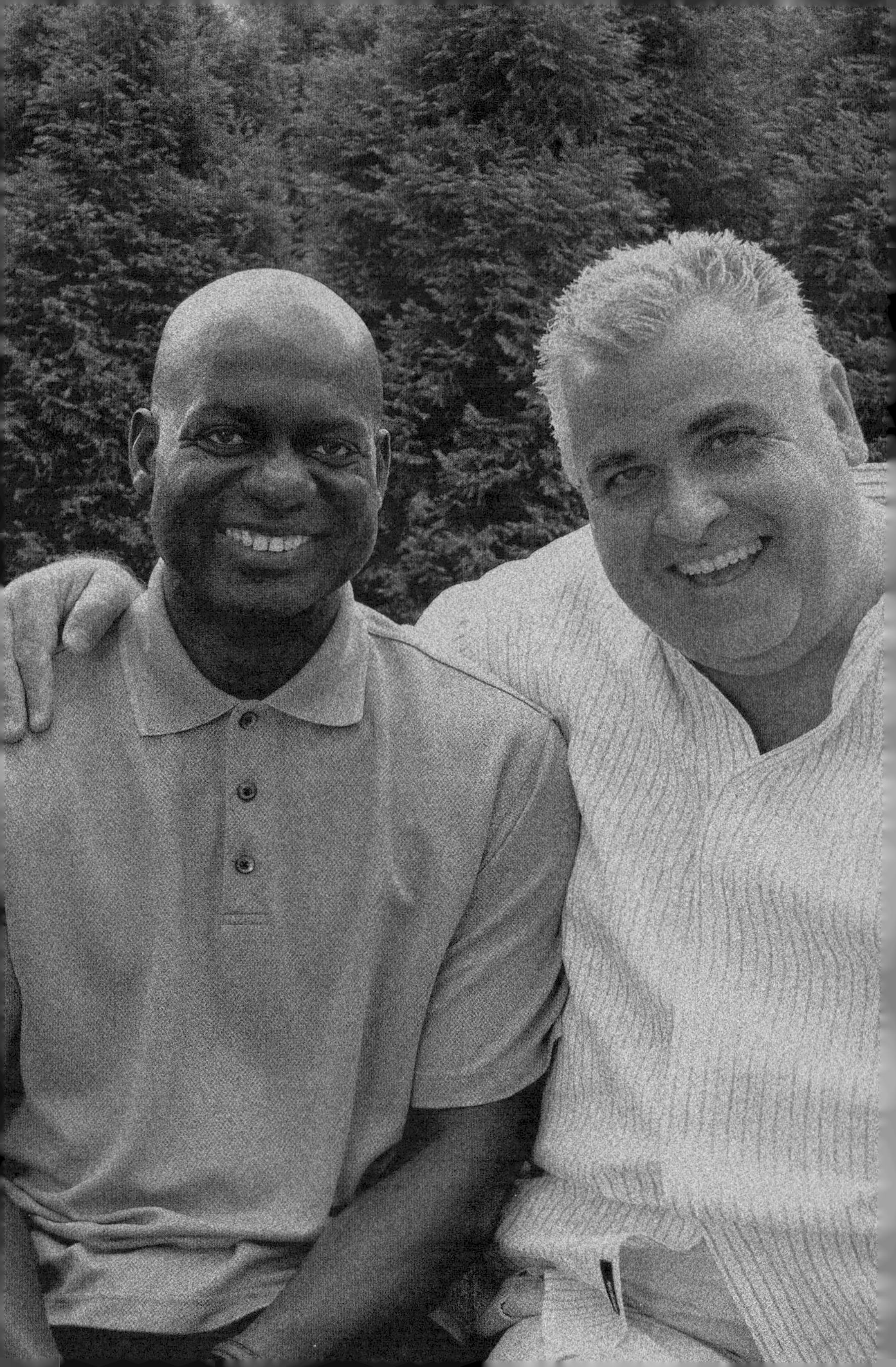

CHAPTER 17

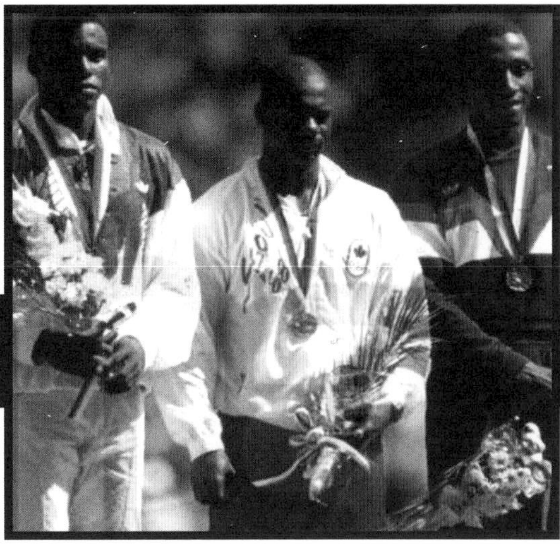

Seoul to Soul

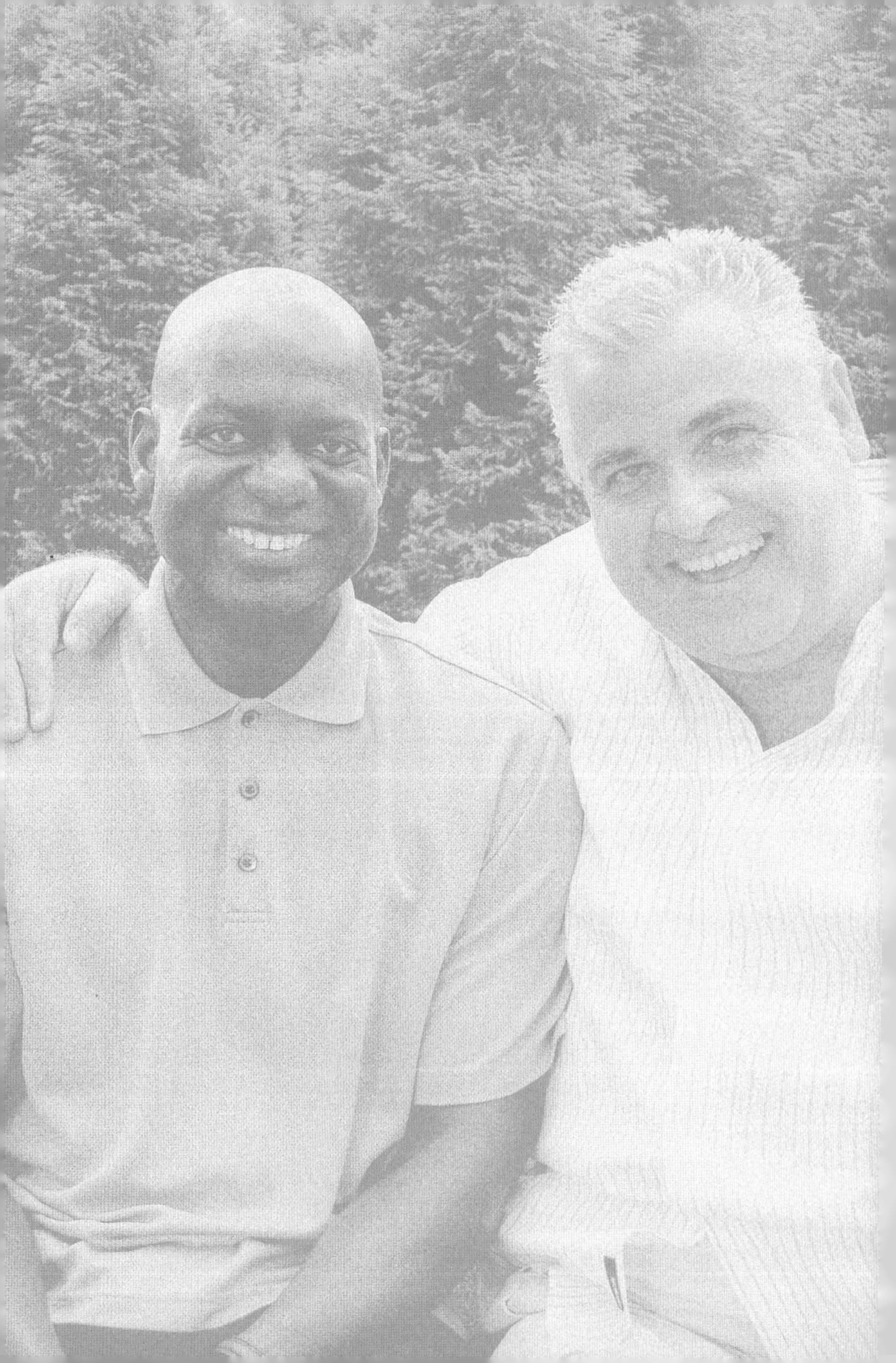

CHAPTER 17

Seoul to Soul

Some in the media have portrayed me as single-handedly destroying the credibility of elite sports and track and field. But many other people continue to believe there is more to my story... there must be. In the last 22 years, I have met so many people around the world who have expressed to me that they always had a gut feeling there was something just not right about the events in Seoul. Many people in politics and the media who were in some way connected to the events surrounding my disqualification know there is more to the story. Most elite athletes, trainers and coaches also suspect, based on their own experiences that there is more than meets the eye to that day in Seoul. At the very least, I would think Carl Lewis suspects this much.

I asked Bryan to discern for me if this is true. God addressed my question:

Ben, you are asking Me again about the feelings of many people... and if many felt you were not treated fairly in Seoul, whether or not they knew, on some level, that you were innocent? Is this not what you are asking?

I responded by nodding my head.

Ben, allow Me to explain to you again. For all of My Children, when each one's spirit and soul come together as one, this is when they will know when Truth has been spoken. So those children of God who have their spirit and soul together as one, it is these children who know without a doubt that you are innocent.

For I say to you, Ben: You have come a long way and I am very proud of you. But remember, those who caused your demise, and those who covered the story of your demise, played a very important role: to allow the world to see how I will take you from being down and out, to a place... to a statue... where you will be walking tall and proud. For you have been able to forgive, and been able to save your soul through the act of forgiveness.

I know that this one 9.79 second event in Seoul, or even the entirety of my career, does not define me. I derive my inner strength from my soul and my faith. My inner strength comes from the faith of those who have always supported me and never gave up on me when the going got tough. My ability comes from my parents' love for me, and my love for them, along with my other family members. Those who know me understand: I was simply a kid who dreamed of running and who did exactly that. I ran with all my heart and soul. And then, I became tarnished by the sport I love.

I asked Bryan to discern if I became tarnished by the sport I love. I looked at Bryan and he began to discern. God spoke:

Ben, so you ask the question, were you tarnished by the sport you love? For I say unto you: Do you truly understand the question that you are asking? Are you deflecting the blame? Are you looking for a shadow? What are you looking for... What are you looking for?

For I know: You are looking for inner peace. For this inner peace will only come when your journey of looking at yourself in the mirror has been completed. We should not blame anyone. We should take full self-accountability and responsibility. Remember: when you were created, you were given the genes to make you run fast, to hold you steady. I have given very few these genes. These genes were given to you... the inner strength came from Me... your inner strength came from Me.

My son, not having a father, I mean your biological father, at your side for you has been difficult. For I know the pain, for I know the burden you have had and that you have overcome. Again, I gave you the inner strength to overcome your pain and your burden. For what you have gone through since Seoul, mentally and emotionally, very few could survive.

I brought you back to Me through Bryan and allowed Bryan to be the vessel to lift the heaviness, the weight from your head and shoulders. My son, through all your struggles I have never turned My back on you. I sent many Messengers to help you. But prior to meeting Bryan, the most important was your mother. She was there for you, to protect you. I say to you, and all My Children: Trust more in My Creation and trust less in man's understanding. For My son, you have asked for forgiveness many times and I have forgiven you.

My son, your mother who you have lost has come back to Me. For I have allowed her to continue in the spirit realm to protect you.

I have learned many truths on my journey. I discovered the most important things in life are faith and family, not material things. I accomplished what I set out to do, whether others choose to acknowledge it or not. My world records were phenomenal and would have stood for 15 years. I thank God for giving me the genes and the inner strength to be successful, and to continue to be successful even though I lost the gold medal.

I will admit, I am disappointed with the manner in which my career ended. But I learned my life's biggest achievement was not running 100 metres in 9.79 seconds. Instead, I learned my biggest achievement was learning to forgive unconditionally. I discovered that education comes in many forms. The life experience I have had taught me not to put my trust in man's world, but instead to trust God. I realized that, unfortunately, jealousy and racism do exist, but there is a reason for everything. I have come to appreciate every day for what it is and live in the now... because life can change drastically in seconds. I believe I have tried to live a good life but more importantly, I know I have lived the life I was supposed to live in order for me to spiritually grow. I have unconditionally forgiven those who harmed me and betrayed my trust. I thank them for the role they played so I could learn to forgive unconditionally and learn to trust God.

With the wisdom of hindsight, I now know I should never have taken steroids at all. They never did help me to run faster. If I had not taken them, I know from my discernments with Bryan, I would have been able to run even faster. If I had another chance, I would definitely not take any steroids or any other kind of drug at all. For anyone who is considering using steroids or any other performance enhancer as part of their track and field training, I would very strongly urge them to reconsider and trust only in how God provided them with the genes to race and all the inner strength they need.

Growing up, my mother demonstrated to my siblings and me a great love of God. Through her own example, she taught us compassion and surrender, to love our neighbour as ourselves and to love God with all our hearts, minds, souls, and strength. In fact, my brother Edward is now a pastor in Texas, serenading the Word of God. My mother always said God is good. I know the future holds good things for me. I am ready to accept whatever God has in store for the second half of my life. I look forward to living a full, healthy and happy life with those who are close to me. I will continue to work with youngsters whom I am able to inspire from time to time, in whatever way this is. I am prepared to be used as an instrument to get God's Truth out to the world.

After the Seoul Olympics, my mother consoled me. She always told me one day it would come to pass that the truth would come out: The events of my life would be clear to all. I know she is correct and that is one reason I chose to publish this book: to fulfill my mother's spiritual discernment. I can see this is now happening for me. I know my mother was spiritually gifted. She was able to discern Truth, on a certain level. She often had visions, like the vision she had in the dream she experienced before my fateful race in Seoul. We both knew these visions she experienced throughout our lives were messages from the Heavens.

In the summer of 2008, I was given the opportunity to meet my spiritual advisor, Bryan Farnum. By trusting in God, I was finally given the chance to confirm and learn a deeper Truth about what happened to me in Seoul and why. As Bryan tells me, the free will we have in life is whether we choose to forgive unconditionally or hold a grudge. That choice comprises the extent of our free will. Through Bryan's gift, I learned that my experience in Seoul was written even before I was conceived and everyone involved was destined to go through it. Knowing there was nothing I could have done to prevent this experience from taking place is a huge relief to me.

After receiving spiritual knowledge and healing through Bryan's gift, I needed to publish this book. I have tried to make my point very clear: My intent is not to seek revenge. Rather, my intent is simply to get the Truth out. The true story turned out to be much bigger than I originally thought! I needed to tell this story from my point of view. By doing this, I forgive everyone involved: I choose to let go and move on in peace. I choose to learn from the life script God has given me. My desire is to transform my story into something truly beautiful. My ultimate intent in publishing this book is to help others who might benefit from my example.

My first appointment with Bryan was an experience I will never forget. I remember the moment I first saw him in his foyer, a handsome, heavyset man standing 6'3" tall and looking like a big teddy bear. His welcoming smile immediately told me, "I'm here to help you." He gave me a big bear hug, as he does with everyone he meets.

I stepped into his office, a healing room. The melody of soft background music touched my soul, softening and opening my heart. The muted tones of sage green walls,

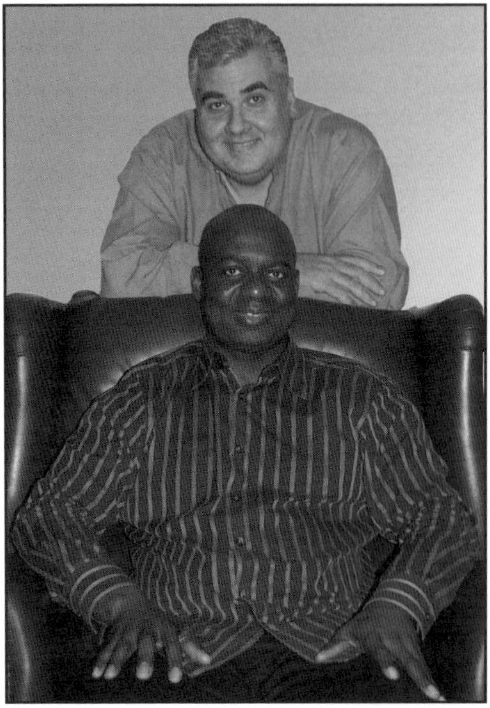

rich leather furniture, and natural light filtering through the window invited me in. I smelled something wonderfully comforting and sweet... frankincense. On the wall, I immediately noticed a painting of Christ standing in the clouds, smiling serenely and hugging a person whose back was toward me. What would it feel like to be that person, embraced by Christ? I wondered.

Bryan sat down on the sofa and invited me to sit in his big leather wing-back armchair. He said he likes to call this chair "the hot seat." He went out of his way to point out, "The reason I'd like you to sit there is because I want you to be comfortable." This is the place where many people have been seated, a place where many healings have taken place. That is the reason why I was there. I was seeking Truth and healing.

In our very first session, I could feel the presence of God. Some call this feeling the Anointing of the Holy Spirit. I felt warmth, even heat, in the room and yet a great sense of calmness and peace. I knew I was in a good place.

What a profound and incredible experience, to just simply sit there and have Bryan discern me. I knew he was seeing me, in my physical body, but he was also looking at my soul. I felt naked and vulnerable, a little scared but safe.

The session began. We spoke about my mother and my father. We spoke about my daughter. We spoke about struggles I've gone through in my life. We spoke about forgiveness. Bryan knew intimate things about me, about my life, without me telling him. He knew things only I knew about myself, things I had never expressed to him or anyone else. He even knew things I did not know about myself. And yet, when he told me these things, part of me knew they were true, even though I had not thought of them before. He told me so many things, things only God could have known.

My first visit with Bryan proved to be an experience I will always treasure for the rest of my life. I know it will be difficult for many to believe there is a person on this planet who knows everyone and they do not have to be in his presence for him to know them. But through his spiritual gift, with permission from God, Bryan really can know everyone, including their ancestors. He can know them so very well.

"The Truth shall set you free," my mother told me. And now here I sat in the hot seat with Bryan, a man who works only for God. He was giving me the Truth, he was helping to set me free. By Bryan presenting me with the spiritual Truth of why certain things happened in my life, I was set free from over 20 years of symptoms of depression. In our very first session, the heaviness, the dark cloud was lifted and my head became very light and clear once again.

Through his gift of discernment, Bryan was able to explain to me some of the reasons why particular struggles were put before me throughout my life, why many of the people in my life had betrayed me. Bryan told me we are all given specific lessons or challenges in our lives. These challenges and struggles are carefully designed. There are no accidents. If we care to examine the so-called "bad" things that happen to us in the right light, we are able to see them as opportunities to spiritually grow. Bryan told me the betrayals of my life were there to help me learn how to forgive unconditionally. I'll admit, throughout my life, this has been a difficult thing for me to do.

Through God's grace that day, I received a discernment verifying what I have always believed was true. Bryan was able to confirm many Truths which have now been revealed in this book. Through this first astounding experience with Bryan, the weight of years and years of anger, sadness, anxiety and symptoms of depression were lifted from me. Through understanding the true reasons why my life unfolded the way it had, I was able to forgive and heal. And through Bryan, I learned the most courageous act a human being can do is to forgive. There is no higher act one can do than to forgive, each other and ourselves. Bryan led me through this process.

First, I needed to ask God to forgive me for whatever I had done throughout my total soul journey which caused me to go through this whole experience of betrayal. Next, I forgave everyone who had harmed me and played a role in my 1988 disqualification where I was stripped of my gold medal and world records. I also needed to forgive my parents for passing away. Each in their own way, they both played such an incredibly supportive role throughout my life and athletic career and I missed them terribly.

But Bryan said we were not yet finished. He told me I needed to forgive myself, perhaps one of the toughest things a person can ever do. Bryan told me one of the main lessons I am supposed to learn in my life is how to overcome being so hard on myself for my setbacks and how to love and forgive myself unconditionally. I needed to understand the true spiritual reasons why I came into this life to have this experience. I had spent the past 20 years punishing myself for letting so many people down. By forgiving myself, I could stop beating myself up. I could heal my soul, reconnect to my heart and reconnect to God.

It was time for me to take accountability and responsibility for my part in the events in Seoul. The biggest mistake I made was to blindly put my trust in man's understanding, rather than to trust in God Who was working through my mother. For this, I now take the opportunity to ask the world to please forgive me.

Bryan gently but confidently guided me through this whole process. I was given the Truth quickly and almost effortlessly. There was no judgment, criticism, blame, guilt, shame, or punishment. There was no need for any of that. All I had to do was surrender to the Truth I was given. I was ready. The entire circumstances of my life experience had all led up to and prepared me for this moment. I was now fully able to accept and embrace the Christ that works through Bryan, keeping in mind that Bryan says Christ is the Spiritual Body of God and lives in the hearts of those who are prepared to receive God.

During and after the healing prayers we said together, I could feel the weight of anger, sadness and anxiety, as well as the heavy symptoms of depression lifting off of me. It was a release I did not realize I needed until it was gone. At that moment, I knew beyond doubt, I had been healed. My head felt light. The heaviness I had been carrying around all these years was gone. It has not returned to this day.

I am so grateful. And I thank God. I give all glory to Him. I thank Bryan for his help and guidance and for serving as the vessel to my healing. I thank my family and everyone else for their support through everything. Through the process of understanding why my life unfolded the way it had, asking for complete forgiveness and completely forgiving everyone, including myself, I have been spiritually set free. Various layers of my soul have been healed. Other layers of my soul are on a continual journey of being healed. I am on a spiritual track.

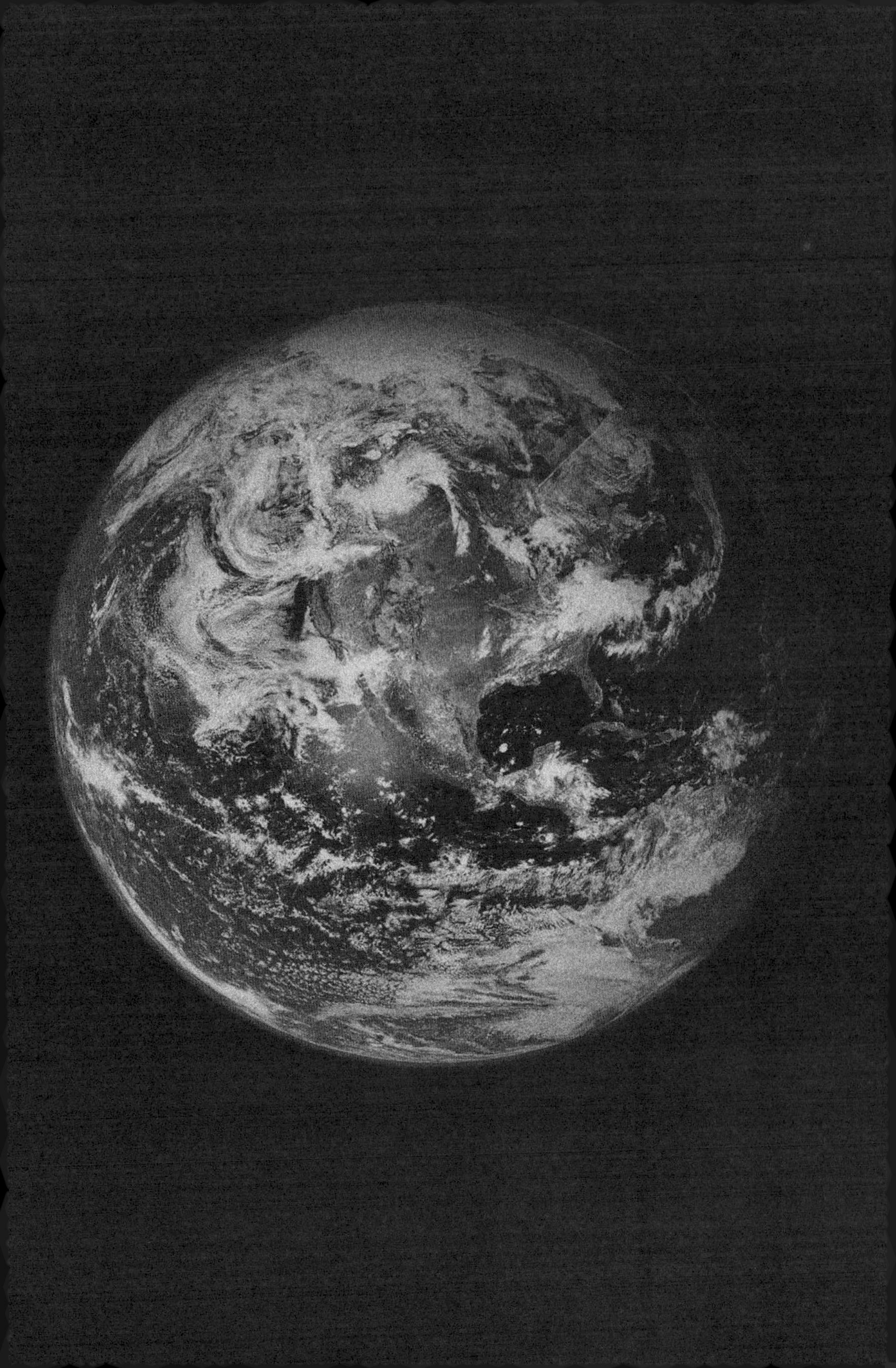

CHAPTER 18

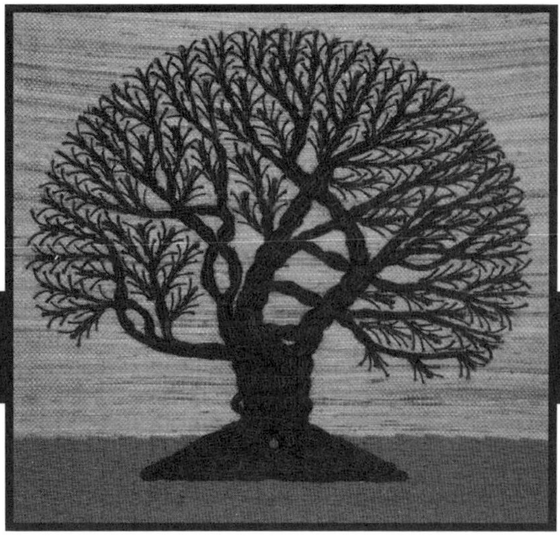

God's Message to the World

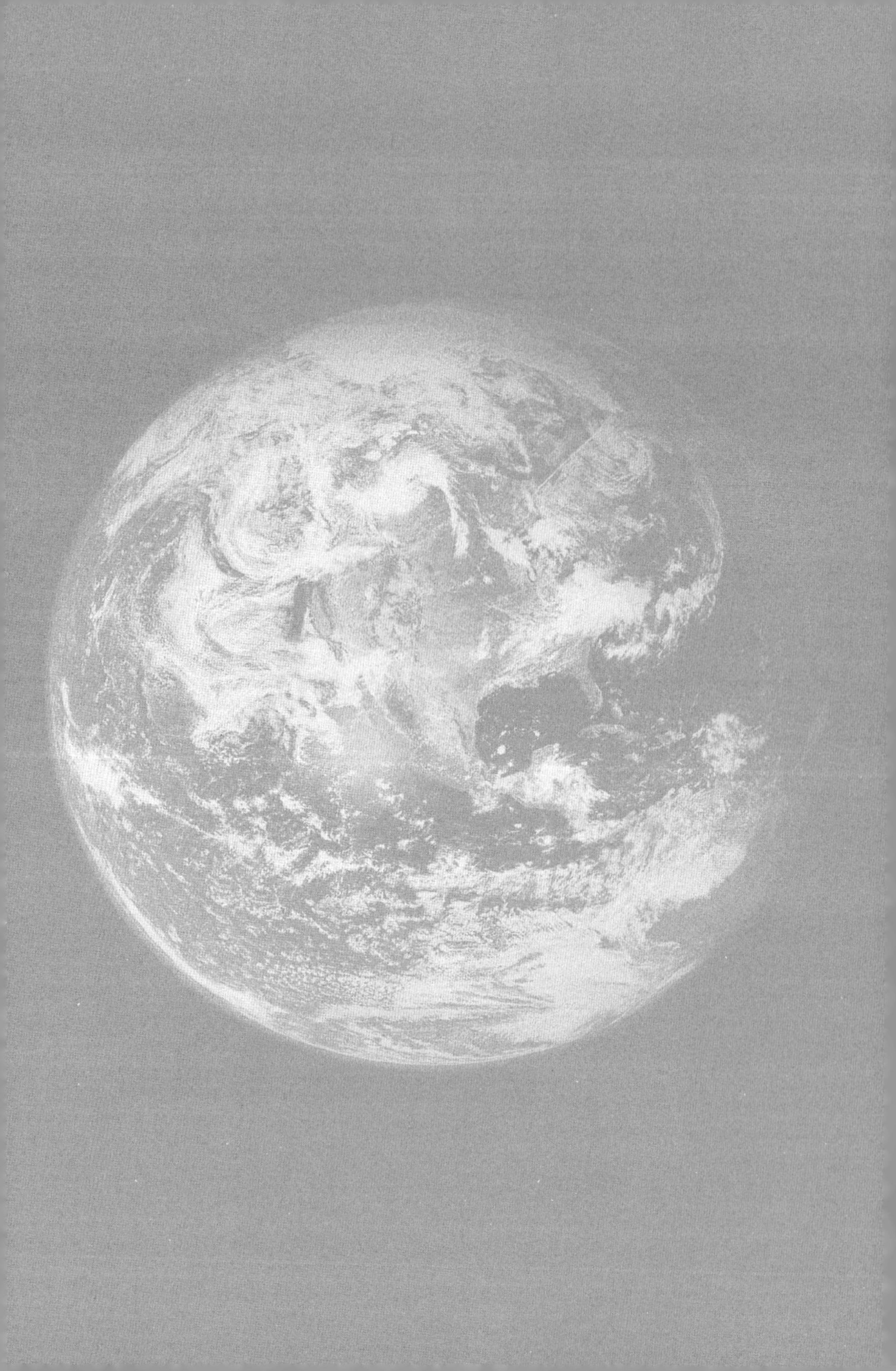

CHAPTER 18

God's Message to the World

My Children, I speak to you through a very brave and courageous Messenger. His name is Bryan Farnum. For I work through Bryan for the world to know Truth... for the world to know Divine Truth.

For all My Children through creation have been given the ability to reconnect to Me. For the process of reconnection shall be long. It shall be challenging for many of you. For some of you will be able to connect to Me in a very short time. For the short time appears to be short. But your conscious does not allow you to recall so easily the many other incarnations you have had that would reveal the incredible long journey you have had.

For I say to all My Children: I am a loving God. I am not a punishing God. For I come to you with One Truth, One Understanding. It is My Will that man, the collective conscious state of man, become a child again and trust only in Me. This process requires all My Children to love and forgive unconditionally. For it is not possible for any of My Children to love Me, to know Me, if My Children do not love themselves or each other.

Throughout time My Children have been misguided. Instead of unity, there is division among My Children. For I have sent One of the Highest, the Only One of the Highest, for His name: My Beloved Son known as Jesus Christ.

For I say unto the world that Bryan was James, brother of Christ. For even back then, in time, some 2,000 years ago, Bryan as James was brave and courageous, for he spoke the Truth without fear. And, for speaking the Truth just like his Brother Jesus, his life was taken. For I have shown Bryan many Truths that are not completely known by all My Children. The Truth around the time of the crucifixion of Jesus Christ... for man at that time was not prepared to become the child again, was not prepared to trust in Me... rather, chose a thief, a murderer, over unconditional love, over unconditional forgiveness.

For My Children chose religions, which are based on many false beliefs. For these false beliefs make Me, the Almighty God, the True Creator to be a punishing God, an unloving God, and an unforgiving God. I say unto all My Children: Do not accept that one must suffer to be with Me. For throughout the universe, it is true that like attracts like.

I am a joyful God. I am a God of the Light. There is no joy found in darkness. I say unto all My Children: I did not make you believe that you must live with guilt and shame, that you are born a sinner, that you will never be worthy to be with Me.

My Children, listen to Me. It is not I who created or encouraged these false beliefs. I am a loving God, a God of unity, a God with many mansions to offer My Children. The possibilities for My Children to have a human experience are vast. For I ask My Children: Do not place limitations on Who God is and what God can do. Do not speak the words, "Oh that is not possible."

Everything is possible.

For I speak of My Children having the experience of more than one incarnation. For I say to all My Children: It is through the false beliefs, it is through the fear... the fear of not wanting to be reminded of the harm that one has done to another, and not wanting to know, to be reminded, of the traumas one may have gone through... It is through false beliefs and fear that many deny the possibility of other incarnations.

Those who deny the possibility of other incarnations, deny self-accountability and self-responsibility.

I ask My Children: Are you one that enjoys seeing people happy? Making others happy? Or are you one that feels very uncomfortable around those who are happy, who are joyful? For My Children: many of My Children have a false belief, if they experience joy, they will be punished by God. My Children, it is My Will for you to experience joy.

It is not My Will for My Children to suffer. It is not My Will for My Children to believe the more that they suffer, the closer to God they become. It is not My Will for the teachings of Armageddon, the end of times, to be taught by anyone to My Children. For those of you who teach Armageddon, the end of times, have anger toward Me. And you have hate towards the world. And you have hate for God's Creation.

I ask all of mankind to come together and learn to love yourself again. Learn to love others again. Learn the Truth that I have to offer to the world through Bryan. Help bring unity to the world and not division.

Many of you who have read this book may be upset with the words written. For in every case, when one has anger, one always has revenge. For I ask My Children who have anger with these words: Who do you have revenge towards?

Just like Ben's heart has been healed, the hearts of My Children can be healed. For I ask all world leaders to agree to an International Forgiveness Day every year, on the fifth month, on the 24th day. Use this opportunity to bring peace among all.

For I say to all My Children: Evil cannot exist without the presence of jealousy. Jealousy cannot exist unless there is some debt that is owing. For the debt is not always recognized. For the debt comes from another time, another incarnation. This is why I have sent Bryan on a mission to help identify the debt among nations, among My People and show all how this debt can be healed and be cleared.

I say to My Children: Do not give away your power. Keep your power by always loving and forgiving unconditionally. For at the very moment you refuse, that you forget to forgive, to forgive another... you have given your power away. For each and every time you hold a grudge... you have given your power away. For how can the Heavens forgive you if you refuse to forgive another?

For what is power? To have power over another, to want power over another, in every case is to have revenge towards another. For My Children, understand: In every case, when one is skeptical, this one does not wish to hear the Truth. This one does not wish to know about common sense. This one believes they must carry out their own revenge. Where does this revenge come from, if the reasoning cannot be identified in this life?

My Children, before you cross over to be with Me: Be free of your anger, of your revenge, of your guilt, of your shame. This surely will come back to create additional challenges in another incarnation.

For many of My Children, when you read this, it will be very difficult for you to accept this. For I will send Bryan throughout the world to help heal My Children and help My Children be free of all false beliefs that prevent My Children from becoming one with Me. For Ben is a walking testimony. For if he refused to believe that this was his only life, today he would still have his symptoms of depression.

I ask My Children: Do not place limitations on God. For those who truly represent Me, they have the ability to discern My Truth on many different levels. For Bryan can discern on a yea, yea; nay, nay basis. And yes, I give him visions. And yes, I come through him effortlessly. My Children, those who are true servants of Mine feel very comfortable with joy, with love, with forgiveness. And they feel very uncomfortable with pain, with suffering, with My Children being misguided.

My Children, for I have already said much. I would also like you to know that I am here to help to reduce the suffering of all My Children. For many, throughout their soul journey, have accepted many false beliefs that suggest the only way to God is by suffering. For I say to all My Children, for this is not so. I am a joyful God, a forgiving God, and a loving God.

For I ask all My Children to stop being so hard on yourself. For there is a danger when one believes that the only way to Me is through suffering. My Children, look before you. Look around. What is the end result, the possible end result of My Children believing they must suffer to come to Me? Will you elect a government leader to bring you joy or to cause you to suffer? If you elect a leader to cause you to suffer, will this leader simply give to you what you're asking? Will this leader maintain peace in your country? With your neighbour? With all other countries? Would your leader protect My Creation? Would your leader support genetically modified foods (GMO)? Would your leader support human cloning? Would your leader support that miracles do not happen? Would your leader support religious false beliefs? Would your leader support military conflict? Would your leader support World War III?

My Children, for I need you to understand very clearly: The false beliefs you hold onto that cause you to believe you must suffer in order to become one with Me, are the same false beliefs that will keep you away from Me and eventually destroy My Creation. For My Children understand: You will elect leaders, support science, based on the belief system that you hold within, that you collectively hold within. For the mirror... for the mirror of your false beliefs will be projected onto others, only to give them permission to bring harm against you and bring suffering against you.

I now ask all My Children: Make a choice... choose to accept your false beliefs and to remain separated from Me... or, be prepared to reject all false beliefs and begin that journey to be one with Me. For I will use Ben as an example to show the world what happens to one when one completely surrenders to Divine Truth.

My Children, I love you.

CHAPTER 19

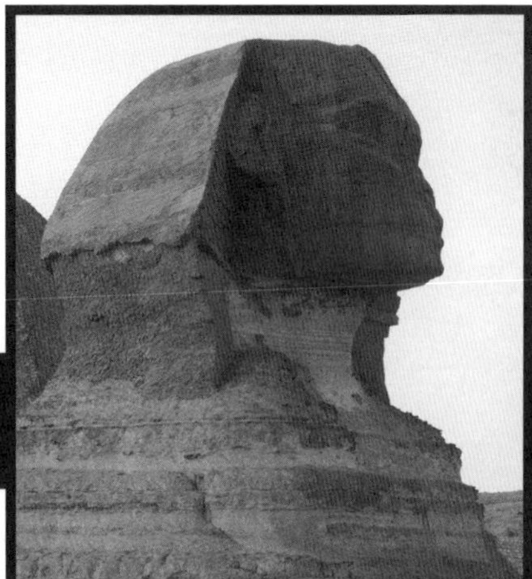

A Message to Ben Johnson from the Lord

CHAPTER 19

A Message to Ben Johnson from the Lord

Ben, My child, I am very proud of you, that you have chosen the path back to Me. For throughout this book, working with Bryan and others, you have asked many questions. For now, I reverse the roles. Now I will give you a Message. And at the end of the Message, I will have one question for you.

For here is My Message to you, Ben... before you came into your mother's womb, you were chosen as a vessel to inspire My Children and to help many of My Children come back to Me. For many of My Children are caught in a web of untruths that hold them hostage, that prevent them from becoming one with Me. I say to you Ben, when one chooses to forgive another, to forgive completely, they in every case choose life. Forgiveness is the primary way how one's soul is cleansed. Forgiveness is an act that requires humility. Forgiveness is an act of resolution. Forgiveness is an act of reducing suffering.

For My Children... as they learn through you, Ben, through this book... for one not to forgive is an act of self-punishment. In every case, when one is not able to forgive another, it is that same reason, same issue that they too have not forgiven themselves for. When they fail to forgive another, they carry the same hatred within themselves.

Ben, in this life, you have suffered much. Much of your suffering goes back to when you were Khufu and you did not forgive. And through subsequent lifetimes, you have suffered. Ben, I am asking you to take this life to end the suffering, to end your suffering, to end the suffering of others around you. For Ben, when you do not forgive, you will attract to yourself that which is unworthy. Many of My Children go to church every day, every week, once a month, once a year, and many, never. If they were able to forgive completely, they would not go to church, for their Temple is within their heart. I do not suggest that My Children do not go to church. For even a church serves a purpose, serves a lesson for one to become, eventually, one with Me.

The human heart has so much influence over the different organs in the body. When the human heart is not completely full of joy, it and many other organs are compromised. When one does not forgive, one chooses dignified suicide. Ben, I say to you: Choose life, and go through life and forgive everyone. The act of forgiveness, Ben, is to benefit you so that one day, you can truly be with Me. For when My Children still have forgiveness to go through, they are not able to have a purpose, a true purpose. And one without a purpose chooses revenge, chooses death. And Ben, for this is profound: The opposite of purpose is always revenge. Ben, seek forgiveness, like you have done, like you continue to do.

Even I need a Purpose to be here with you, to teach My Children and help My Children. Ben, in every case, when one has to forgive another, one is disconnected from Me. And when one is disconnected from Me, one is not able to know Truth, even when Truth has been revealed.

For it is not possible for you or anyone else to have true hope if one still has to forgive another. For if one still has to forgive another, one is truly not able to love unconditionally. One is not truly able to love oneself. And if one is truly not able to love oneself, one is not able to love Me, to love others.

For when My Children do not forgive another, this is where they wish power over another. This is where they wish to fulfill revenge on some level. But I say to you, Ben, and to all My Children: if one is not able to forgive completely, they will experience a shorter human life; they will increase physical suffering for themselves and even for others. For when they are not able to truly forgive, they are not able to truly experience joy. Too many of My Children live a life of fantasy. They live a life of fantasy, fear of knowing Truth. For many of My Children, through this life of fantasy, present a phony image to others, lacking sincerity, only to exact at that right moment, their revenge. For they will justify their actions and will not admit their intentions.

For Ben, I will be with you. I will stay with you. I am not a punishing God. I am not a God that needs My Children to suffer to be with Me. For My Children, if you have not completely forgiven all, you will not take self-accountability and self-responsibility. You will blame others. You may even blame Me. I ask My Children to forgive all and do not take satisfaction in seeing others suffer.

Ben, I know I've given you a deep Message, a lengthy Message, and you can see from what has been revealed to you why it is important for you to forgive André Jackson, Carl Lewis, everyone... yourself, remembering that the benefit of complete forgiveness mostly goes in your favour. My child, I do not wish to see you suffer another lifetime. I do not wish you to create more karma for yourself by not going through the complete forgiveness journey. For I need you to be with Me. I need you to inspire My Children. I need you to become the child again. For this is how you must be, to be with Me. For those of My Children who will not accept this Message, the Message that has been revealed to you, for you to accept in its entirety... for those children who do not accept this Message will likely enter into a soul journey of darkness, a journey of suffering, a journey of not knowing Truth, a journey with those of empty hearts.

My question to you, Ben: are you with Me?

We are all on a soul journey and mine has not been easy. From the time of my soul's inception, I ask all to forgive me for bringing any harm against them. I thank all who played a role to facilitate the soul journey I experienced. Through my relationship with God, I do know that God is real and that all things are possible once we forgive. Thank You, Father. And yes, I am with You.

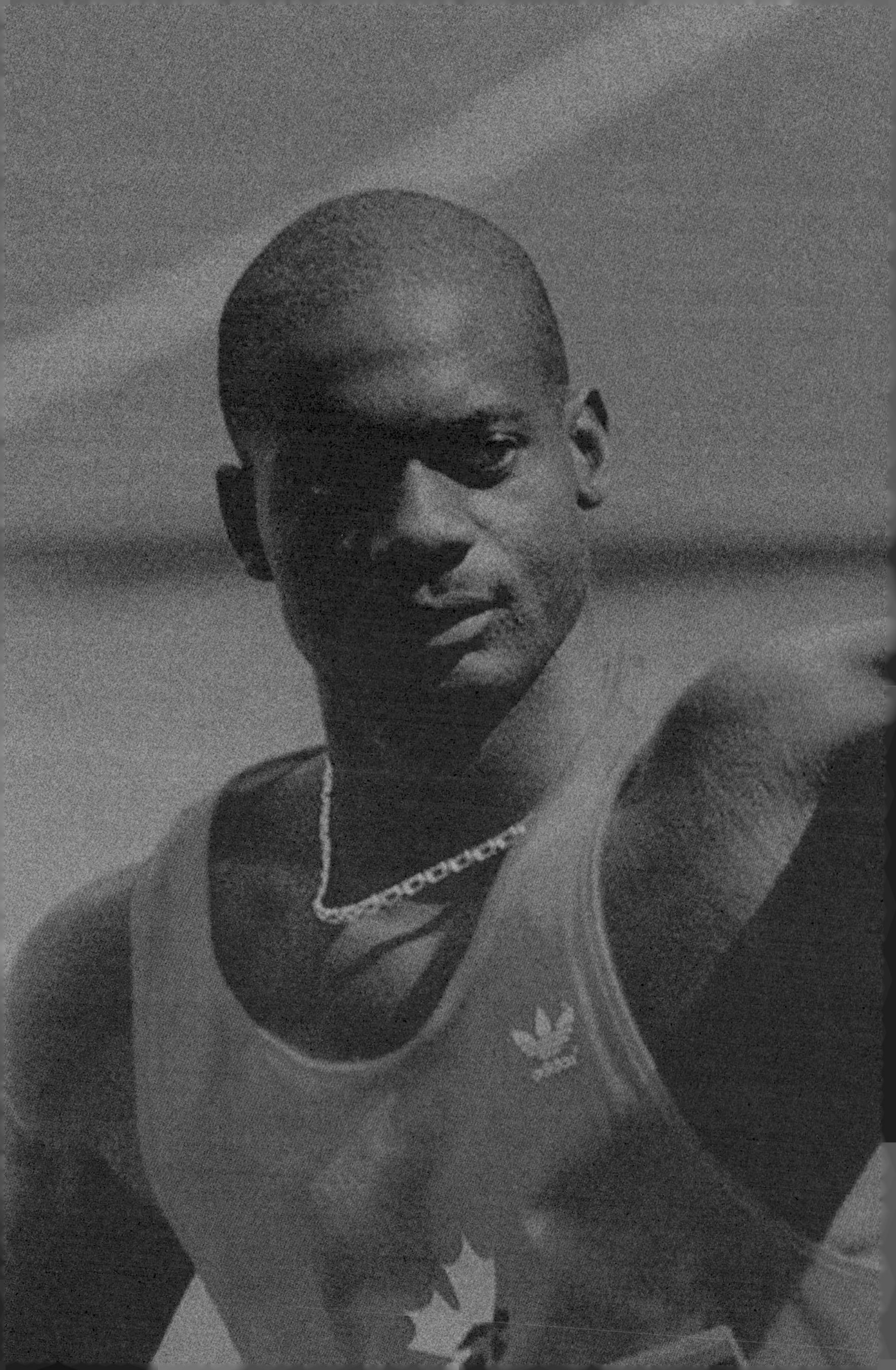

CHAPTER 20

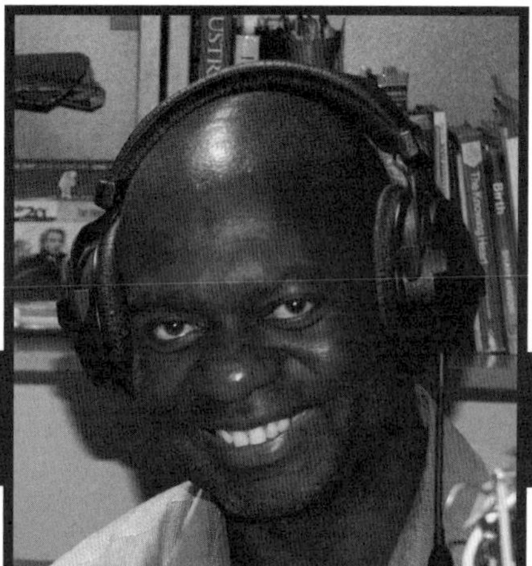

Questions I Always Wanted to Ask God About My Life

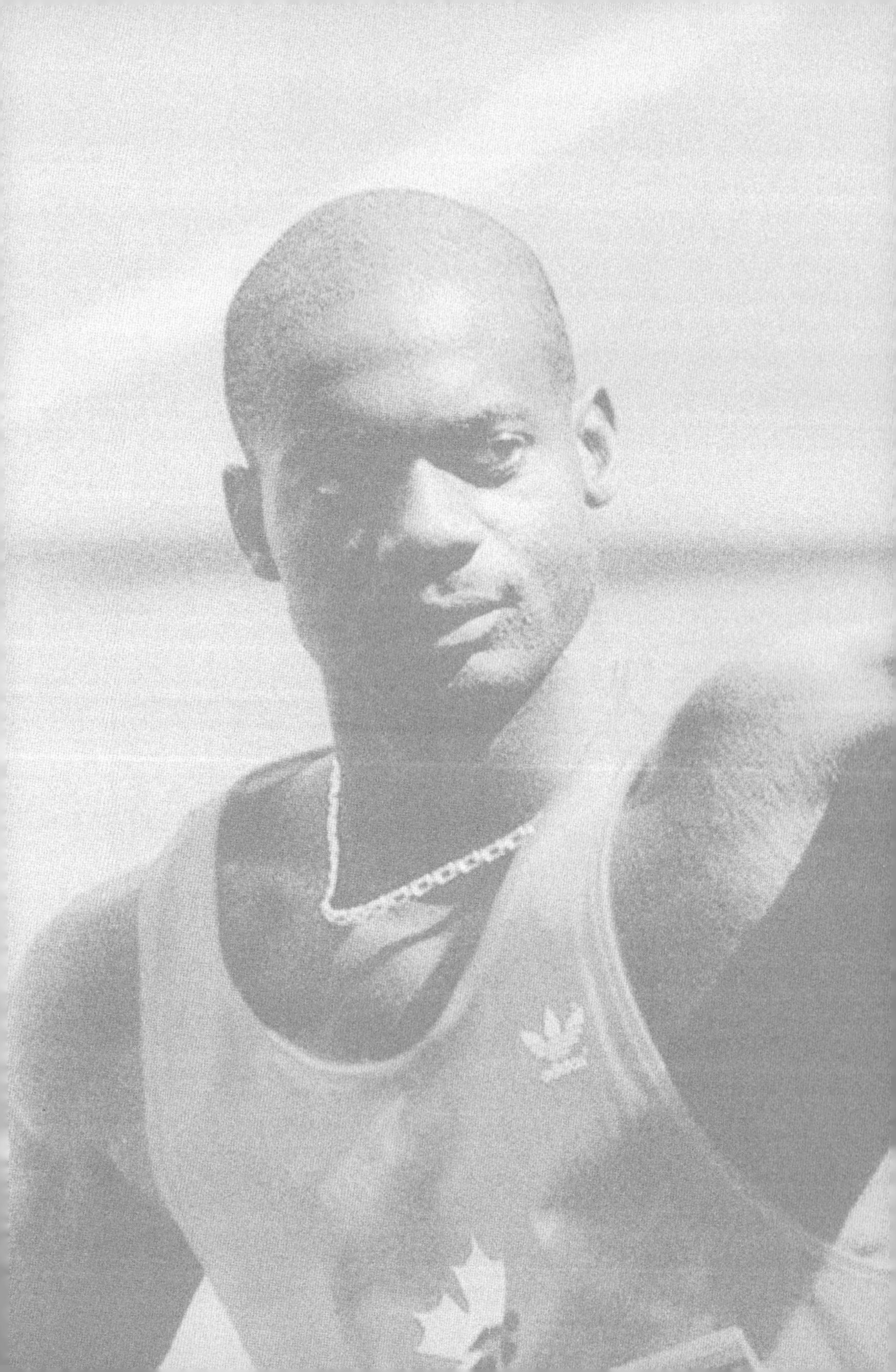

CHAPTER 20

Questions I Always Wanted to Ask God About My Life

After the final race in Seoul, so many people noticed and commented on the fact that I did not smile. After the scandal broke, many wondered if this was a sign that I knew I did not win the race fairly. This insinuation always bothered me. I was so happy in my heart that day. It did not make sense to me that they said I was not smiling. But on review of film and photographs taken that day, I have to admit, I can see their point. So, the first question I asked God was, why did I not smile at the medal award ceremonies in Seoul?

Bryan sat back in his chair and closed his eyes. He surrendered himself to God and began to speak:

Ben, you ask the question... many have asked the question, why were you not joyful? Why was this not clearly evident by a smile from you when you received the gold medal at the 1988 Seoul Award Ceremonies? For the answer will not be accepted by many. The answer will be very difficult for many to understand. But, most of My Children come into each incarnation with spirits that influence their overall behaviour, that influence the experience that they are to have.

At the moment you received the gold medal, a spirit took charge of you. And this spirit prevented you from smiling. For the spirit came from another incarnation, based on a religious false belief, a distorted belief, on how one should give Me, God, the glory.

For this spirit did not give you free will. It forced you to give Me the glory. This is not God's Will. For My Children should have much more free will. But these spirits that hold them hostage from other incarnations have taken away most of My Children's free will.

For I ask My Children: The only way to give Me true glory is to live according to the two suggested commandments of God. And most of My Children know what these commandments are. Because of the false beliefs religion teaches, and other influences, My Children have a difficult time accepting, understanding, and living according to these two suggested commandments. For they are: Love God with all your heart, soul, mind and strength... and that means not to blame God and not to believe that I am a punishing God and to take full self-accountability and responsibility for one's own actions, or lack of action... I have suggested to My Children through many Messengers to love thy neighbour as thyself... and that means, to do no harm to another, to love another, to forgive another, and to bring unity among all and not division.

Ben, as Bryan is the vessel, he will lift this spirit from you. He will set you free from the false belief that you should be forced to give Me glory, that you should have guilt because you received the gold medal. For you will be set free from this spirit. And I ask you and all My Children: From this moment on, live according to the two suggested commandments. And Ben, continue on your spiritual journey and cleanse your soul and remove the other spirits of false belief to completely set yourself free. I ask My Children, all My Children to follow a similar path.

I said to Bryan, "I would like to get that spirit off me as soon as possible. Let's do it after all my questions have been answered! Is that okay, Bryan?"

"Of course," Bryan laughed, "we have lots of time. Where are we going at this moment, eh?" Then Bryan looked at me and asked me what my next question was.

Next I asked about the people who helped me throughout my running career. In one of my private sessions with Bryan, he discerned that many who helped me are very angry because they lost an opportunity to make a lot of money when the scandal broke out in Seoul. My question was, why did they come into my life to have such an experience? God replied:

Ben, I will answer your question and it will be short. It will be a short answer. For it is wise for one to have no expectations. For My Children must understand: Those who are highly successful, who are highly successful through Me, they are successful because they have no expectations. It is true: The greater the expectation, the more unlikely that one will succeed. But with many of those who were close to you throughout your career and who are still angry, for they too are on a spiritual journey. And they too will go through different experiences to successfully complete, to master, certain spiritual lessons. Many of those whom we speak of who are angry, for they did not truly lose money. They gained. They gained by paying off a spiritual debt that was owed to you from another incarnation, from other incarnations. And, they should rejoice that their debt has been paid to you.

When I heard this response, I had to confirm with Bryan, "So those who we speak of, do I have any spiritual debt still remaining to them?" Bryan responded immediately, "God, the God who is in your heart, says, *Your spiritual debt that you speak of... for there is no more debt. You have been set free.*"

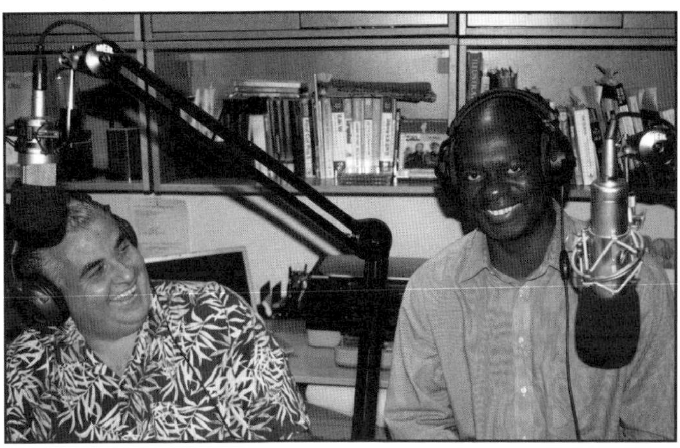

So, my next question... I looked at Bryan and I asked, "Why me? Why you? Why are we together in this lifetime?"

Ben, in a prior session with Bryan, it was revealed to you. For Bryan, in at least ten other incarnations, separate incarnations, was your father, your biological father. This is one reason why you have come together. Bryan has much love for you, just as he has much love for all of My Children. But does he not speak to you like a father? Does he not look out for you? For I have brought both of you together on a very important mission: to bring My People, My Children back to Me.

"Thanks Dad," I laughed.

"It is true. You are a joker! There is humour in you, Ben."

"Now, Dad... just kidding, Bryan... could you please discern for me, how does one know that God is working through you?" I couldn't wait to hear God's answer.

Ben, so you ask the question... the question really is... is Bryan of the Light? Is he a true Messenger of God? When I say God, we speak of the Divine God of Light, of Truth, of Unconditional Love, of Unconditional Forgiveness. We do not speak of false gods, gods of distortion, gods of deception, gods of division.

My son, you have had many opportunities to know Bryan, to know that God is working... that God is working, that I am working through Bryan. Would you be so joyful today and so hopeful today if your spirit of depression was not lifted? The answer is no. Bryan speaks of love. He speaks of unity. He speaks of peace. He speaks. Many listen. Many ignore. And many judge. For those who reject Bryan, reject Me... reject Truth. They have anger, they have revenge in their hearts. They are separated from Me and they have become their own god. They have become their own punishing god. You will know Bryan, the world will know Bryan through his works. He is not afraid to sit down with the President of the United States, the Queen of England, the Prime Minister of Canada, the Pope, the world... as he mentions on his radio broadcast, the 50 cameras... For he is not afraid to have a debate, whether the topic is on religion, on science, on life, on Me, on the universe, on anything. He is not afraid. But most are afraid to sit with Bryan. Because their soul knows, they are part of a Math Equation that knows when Truth has been delivered, they cannot hide behind the cloak of their false beliefs.

I say to all My Children: Embrace Divine Truth, embrace Me, and let go of all false beliefs that make you believe you must suffer. For the teachings that My Children must suffer to get to Me, to be with Me, is not of Me.

I was still and speechless. There were no further questions to be asked.

Then Bryan spoke these words to me:

From this moment on, when God's Children see your face, your face will symbolize:

- endurance
- determination
- respect
- that you are open to the world
- that you provide God's Children with hope.

That is what your face, your name symbolizes.

Thank You, Father.

Ben, I will give you a new purpose. And this purpose will be profound. And I will use you as a vessel to bring joy to My Children. For what you have lost, I will give it back to you. But you must remember, all My Children must remember: If you have a purpose, you choose life. If you lose your purpose or have no purpose, you choose death. My Purpose is to provide Truth to My Children, to My Creation. I ask My Children: Allow Me with great joy to continue to fulfill My Purpose.

I asked, "Is it true that mankind will remain as long as man does not turn his back on God, for God to lose His Purpose with man?"

And Bryan looked at me with sadness and responded, "Yes."

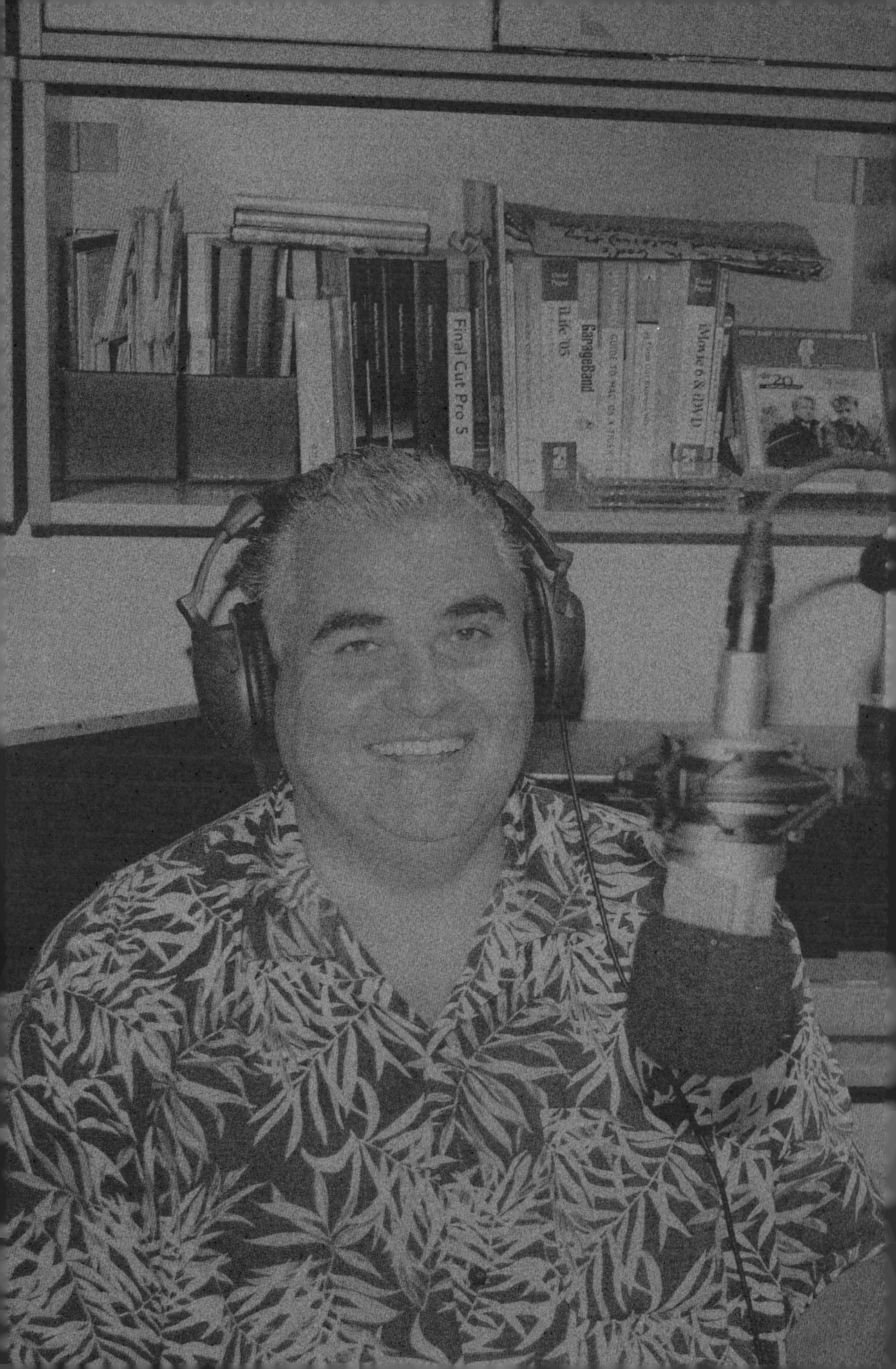
Final Cut Pro 5
iLife '05
GarageBand

WORDS OF WISDOM

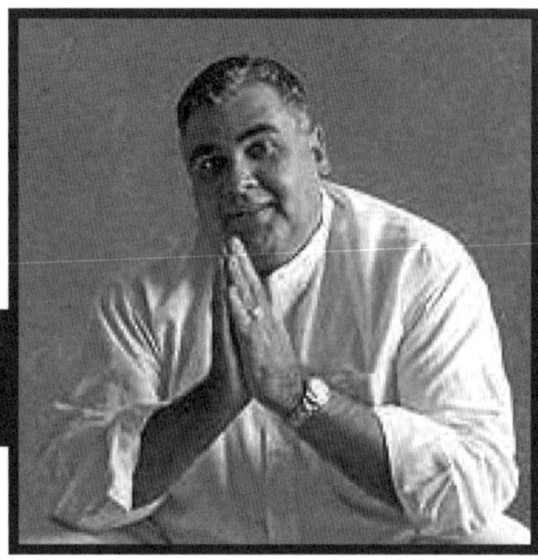

by Bryan Farnum

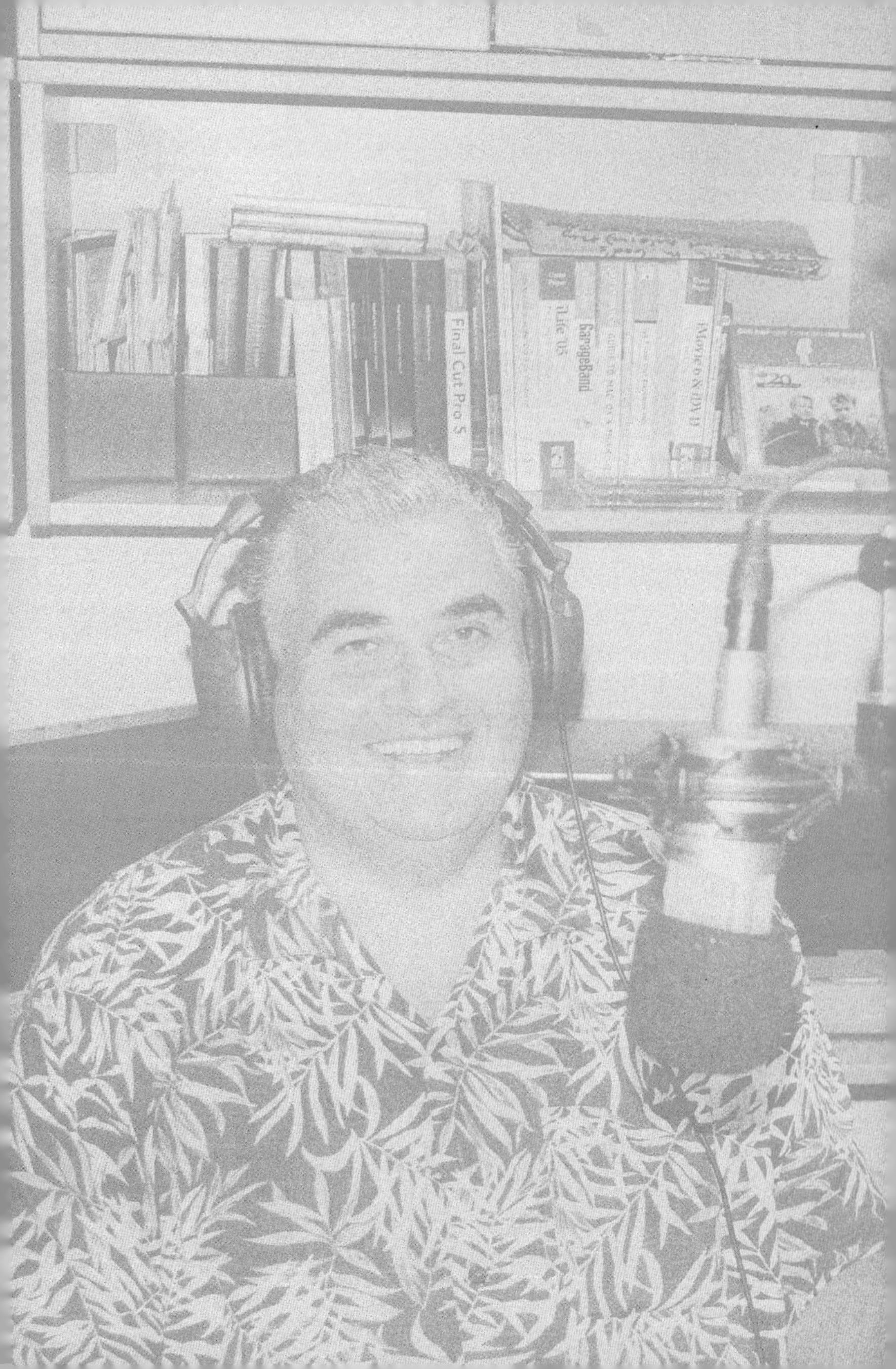
Final Cut Pro 5
GarageBand
iLife 05

Words of Wisdom by Bryan Farnum

The life journey for many of us is not so easy, especially when compared to others who seem more fortunate. Many of our life circumstances are based on experiences we may have had in other incarnations. Religion places limitations on God and refuses to accept personal self-accountability and self-responsibility. Refusal to accept accountability and responsibility is the main reason why many in religion do not believe they may have had another incarnation. This refusal results in the character attribute of skepticism. Skepticism prevents people from knowing Truth and prevents them from being able to forgive others or even themselves.

A skeptic is not allowed to have common sense. This is because by accepting Truth, it prevents the skeptic from fulfilling their own revenge on another. There is not one skeptic who has a heart free of revenge. So, in most cases, those who will speak against Mr. Ben Johnson are speaking as a result of their own revenge they may have towards him, or their own revenge they have towards themselves.

Many people will call another evil. But evil cannot exist if jealousy does not exist. For evil is how one reacts to jealousy. For one to call another evil, they are judging that person, so therefore they are judging themselves. They are calling themselves evil. It is only when our soul has been completely cleansed, we will only see good in another.

In the case of Ben Johnson, throughout this life, and throughout other incarnations, many have become very jealous of him. This jealousy has turned into anger and then into revenge, only to achieve the final result of skepticism. It is important that the world understands this. On a micro level, jealousy can come between athletes in competition, creating intense rivalry. And then, on a macro level, jealousy can come between one nation and another nation. In every case, jealousy, if left unchecked, can destroy a person, can destroy a nation. And, eventually within this universal matrix that we are all part of, jealousy will always destroy the one who is jealous.

What you sow, you shall reap. The only answer to offset jealousy is to apply forgiveness and remove greed from the collective consciousness of humankind. We must always remember: The only currency in the spirit world is forgiveness. When we are completely free of jealousy, we will be completely free of many false beliefs. One such false belief, for example, is the Old Testament adage of "an eye for an eye", the belief that we must act out our revenge on another for what has been done to us, getting even. It is not possible for religions to exist once all the false beliefs have been removed from mankind's consciousness. False beliefs only keep us in bondage, like a rat on a treadmill. When the treadmill stops, the rat has made no progression. It is still standing in the exact same spot.

At the end of the day, it takes a very courageous person to forgive and it takes a coward to act out their own revenge. To be one with God, one must be free of all judgment. In every case, when one judges another, one is judging themselves. For the same weakness they see in others, they also, in every case, have the same weakness within themselves.

Touch not My anointed

and do those who serve Me no harm.

PHOTO CREDITS

I would like to thank everyone who contributed pictures to the book:

Claus Anderson, Dust jacket back cover foreground and background, Dust jacket inside left flap (top), Dedication left side, Preface, pages 2, 3, 4, 5, 24, 25, 26, 34, 38, 43, 98, 99, 100, 113, 116, 117, 118, 123, 134, 135, 136, 138, 139, 146, 150, 152, 159, 186, 187, 188, 193, 195, 213, 238, 240.

Val Grosse, pages 84, 86.

Stewart R. Leslie, pages 232, 233, 234.

Waldemar Matuszewski, pages 57, 151, 162.

Donald Quarrie, page 112.

Sun Media, pages 14, 15, 16, 20, 42, 44, 46, 49, 56, 58, 68, 142, 143, 144, 155, 174, 175, 176, 179, 205, 210.

CAPTIONS

Front cover Me, now

Back cover Me, back in the mid-eighties
In the background, running the 100 metre final in Seoul

Inside left flap 100 metre final in Seoul
My grand-daughter Micaila and me

Dedication Rome 1987
My mother Gloria and me

Preface Crossing the finish line in Seoul 1988, breaking the world record, in 9.79 seconds

Chapter 1 – Winning the Race but Losing My Medal

Page 2, 4 Rome 1987
Page 3 Taken in Seoul, arranging my singlet
Page 5 Shortly after crossing the finish line after the final race in Seoul

Chapter 2 – What Happened?

Page 14, 16 My mother and me arriving in Toronto after Seoul
Page 15 The car picking us up at Pearson, surrounded by media
Page 20 The media camped in front of my house in the aftermath of Seoul.

Chapter 3 – Performance-Enhancing Steroids

Page 24, 26 A training session for Seoul at York University Track
Page 25 Doing 150m repeats in a training session for Seoul at York University Track
Page 34 Carrying the torch into Toronto for the 1988 Winter Olympic Games
Page 38 In Rome

Chapter 4 – The Dubin Inquiry

Page 42, 44 My lawyer and me arriving at the Dubin Inquiry
Page 43 On the witness stand at the Dubin Inquiry
Page 46 Well-wishers from Winston Churchill School showing support
Page 49 Among the media after the Dubin Inquiry

Chapter 5 – "The Mystery Man" Comes Forward

Page 56, 58 Well-wishers showing support in front of my house
Page 57 Carl Lewis and André Jackson in the doping testing area in Seoul
Page 68 My mother, Gloria, and me

Chapter 11 – Being the Fastest Man on Earth

Page 142, 144 Driving my Ferrari on the 401
Page 143 Some of my awards
Page 146 Carl Lewis shaking my hand after the final in Rome 1987

Chapter 12 – Fame and Injury

Page 150, 152 Being interviewed after a race, with my mother beside me
Page 151 Receiving treatment from Waldemar
Page 155 Washing my Ferrari
Page 159 Carrying the Canadian flag at the Opening Ceremonies in Edinburgh 1986
Page 162 Receiving treatment from Waldemar

Chapter 13 – The Calm Before the Storm

Page 166, 168 On vacation
Page 167 Dr. Jamie Astaphan and my mother
Page 170 At the beach
Page 171 Enjoying boating

Chapter 14 – On to Seoul

Page 174, 176 The flight to Seoul
Page 175 Warm up track in Seoul, drinking from a water bottle from the tent
Page 179 Charlie and me arriving in Seoul

Chapter 15 – The Chaos of Champions

Page 186, 188 Semifinal in Seoul
Page 187 Winning the Gold Medal Race in Seoul
Page 193 Reviewing the scoreboard in Seoul... will I make it into the next round?
Page 195 Reaction to being called for a false start... which it wasn't...